STILL
DOWN

STILL
DOWN

What to Do When Antidepressants Fail

Dean F. MacKinnon, MD

Johns Hopkins University Press
Baltimore

Note to the Reader: This book is not meant to substitute for medical care of people with *mental disorders*, and treatment should not be based solely on its contents. Instead, treatment must be developed in a dialogue between the individual and his or her physician. This book has been written to help with that dialogue.

Drug dosage: The author and publisher have made reasonable efforts to determine that the selection of drugs discussed in this text conform to the practices of the general medical community. The medications described do not necessarily have specific approval by the US Food and Drug Administration for use in the diseases for which they are recommended. In view of ongoing research, changes in governmental regulation, and the constant flow of information relating to drug therapy and drug reactions, the reader is urged to check the package insert of each drug for any change in indications and dosage and for warnings and precautions. This is particularly important when the recommended agent is a new and/or infrequently used drug.

© 2016 Johns Hopkins University Press
All rights reserved. Published 2016
Printed in the United States of America on acid-free paper
9 8 7 6 5 4 3 2 1

Johns Hopkins University Press
2715 North Charles Street
Baltimore, Maryland 21218-4363
www.press.jhu.edu

Library of Congress Cataloging-in-Publication Data

Names: MacKinnon, Dean F., author.
Title: Still down : what to do when antidepressants fail / Dean F. MacKinnon.
Description: Baltimore : Johns Hopkins University Press, 2016. | Series: A johns hopkins press health book
Identifiers: LCCN 2016005166| ISBN 9781421421056 (hardcover) | ISBN 1421421054 (hardcover) | ISBN 9781421421063 (paperback) | ISBN 1421421062 (paperback) | ISBN 9781421421070 (electronic) | ISBN 1421421070 (electronic)
Subjects: LCSH: Depression, Mental—Treatment—Popular works. | Antidepressants—Popular works. | BISAC: SELF-HELP / Depression. | PSYCHOLOGY / Psychopathology / Depression. | MEDICAL / Psychiatry / General.
Classification: LCC RC537 .M318 2016 | DDC 616.85/27—dc23
LC record available at https://lccn.loc.gov/2016005166

A catalog record for this book is available from the British Library.

Special discounts are available for bulk purchases of this book. For more information, please contact Special Sales at 410-516-6936 or specialsales@press.jhu.edu.

Johns Hopkins University Press uses environmentally friendly book materials, including recycled text paper that is composed of at least 30 percent post-consumer waste, whenever possible.

CONTENTS

TABLES

ACKNOWLEDGMENTS

I offer sincere gratitude to many friends, colleagues, and patients who encouraged me to write this book, and who read and commented on the text as I was writing it. In particular, I thank my wife, Dr. Catherine Washburn, Drs. Ray DePaulo and John Dougherty, along with Barbara Schweizer, Sunny Mendelsohn, and Dr. Eileen Epstein. Finally, the book owes its existence to the many patients who have shared not only their symptoms but also their life stories with me.

STILL
DOWN

Introduction

Major depressive disorder is among the most common and
debilitating medical conditions. The illness can hang on for
months, even years, and annually drives about a million people
to suicide around the world. Its biological mechanisms are
uncertain, so no medicine can fix the cause of the problem.
Anyone unfortunate enough to have one episode of major
depressive disorder is likely to have more episodes, throughout life.

Although incurable, major depression is highly treatable. In
the middle of the twentieth century, pharmacologists discovered
that several drugs developed for other medical problems,
taken daily, could reverse the symptoms of major depressive
disorder within six to eight weeks. Dozens of other antidepressant drugs that have similar pharmacologic effects have been
invented since that time. About two of every three people who

have major depression and who take a sufficiently strong dose of an antidepressant daily for six to eight weeks will experience a significant reduction in the symptoms of depression. For those who had either no response or an incomplete response, a switch to one of the many other antidepressants approved by the US Food and Drug Administration may bring relief. But even people who do experience a satisfactory response remain at high risk for relapse. Psychiatrists have worked out a variety of medication tricks to boost response and avert relapse. Psychotherapy helps, too. For the most severely afflicted, electroconvulsive therapy can be lifesaving. The painfully slow search for better and safer treatments continues, occasionally yielding a promising new method to alleviate depression.

My primary clinical role as a psychiatrist for the past twenty-odd years in both inpatient and outpatient settings has been to try to help people who have not responded adequately to treatment for depression. The key to my approach is to focus on a question all too seldom asked: Why did the standard treatment not work for this person? This book uses nine patient stories to illustrate how I try to understand and help people who have failed to respond to antidepressant treatment. Let me assure the patients I have treated or consulted with that any resemblance between them and these composite cases is purely coincidental.

The stories that follow illustrate some of the ways antidepressant treatment often goes awry. The plan of the book is to progress from the easiest to the hardest cases. The easiest cases are those in which the person has simply not had adequate treatment, so the first section discusses the standard approaches to effective antidepressant treatment and common obstacles to achieving it: overly conservative dosing, not adhering to treatment, and other impediments to adequate therapy, such as high sensitivity to side effects.

The second section looks at misdiagnosis: people who feel and appear depressed but do not presently have major depressive disorder and so cannot be expected to respond well to antidepressants. Flaws within our diagnostic rules and methods often lead clinicians to diagnose major depression in people who are merely demoralized by life circumstances; people who have manias or hypomanias (milder manias) in addition to major depressive episodes, hence exhibiting some form of bipolar disorder; and people who have depressive symptoms while in a state of delirium or intoxication, that is, a disruption of consciousness because of gross, global abnormality in brain function (some might call this "organic" depression).

The third section looks at the cases that experts would classify truly as "treatment resistant" or "treatment refractory." Here there is no doubt about the potential usefulness of antidepressants or about the person's poor response to standard treatments. Some of these patients once had major depressive disorder and responded partially to treatment but have not returned to their previous level of function. Some continue to have a clear major depressive syndrome despite fully adequate medication choices and levels.

Throughout each story, the reader will find numbered links to commentary that explains, extends, or discusses the point being made in the case vignette. Read independently of the case vignettes, this commentary serves as a brief and general survey of the common obstacles to effective antidepressant treatment and of strategies to overcome them.

In this book there are few references to specific medications. In most cases it does not matter which antidepressant the person was or should be using. Antidepressant efficacy is more or less the same across medications, and because individual response is variable, I do not want to be perceived as advertising a particular agent. When I do refer to a specific medication by name, it is because it has some property that makes it unique among its peers. The therapeutic practices described are not thoroughly "evidence-based" in the sense that all have passed muster through controlled clinical trials. Evidence-based approaches are most valuable when the treating professional has limited information about the individual patient and the likelihood that the patient will respond to standard treatment. All else equal, knowing nothing except the diagnosis and treatment response, an evidence-based approach might provide a probabilistic rationale to try one drug over another, or to refer for psychotherapy sooner rather than later. But knowing more about the complicating factors of temperament, behavior, and situation that contribute to treatment failure informs an individualized approach that allows the clinician to avoid educated guesswork and work directly toward treating the patient's problems.

As a way to help the reader keep track, I have assigned names for each fictional patient and clinician that start with the letter of the alphabet that corresponds to the order of the stories. So case 1 is Ann, whose physician is Dr. Abernathy; case 2 is Bob, who is treated by Dr. Beasly; and so on.

This book may be of particular interest to four sorts of reader. For people who have depression, bipolar disorder, or another mental disorder—and their loved ones—I hope that the cases might prompt a more fruitful conversation with the treating physician or practitioner about why the drugs don't work. To primary care providers, who do the majority of antidepressant treatment, the book may help resolve some clinical problems without the need to refer for specialty help or, alternatively, inform a decision about whether a psychotherapist, a general psychiatrist, or a mood disorder specialist might be the best care provider to whom a challenging patient should be referred. Psychotherapists may gain some new insight from this book into the interplay of brain and mind in the expressions of low mood. And for my psychiatric colleagues, I hope these cases may reframe the problem of antidepressant failure from "Which drug will work better?" to "Is another drug really the best treatment for this person's depression?"

I : FUNDAMENTALS

These three stories illustrate the standard approach to treating major depression and a few common obstacles to adequate treatment.

ANN

Textbook Depression

• •

OVERVIEW: Ann's life has been upended by an episode of major depressive disorder. She has most of the classic signs and symptoms. Her primary care physician recognizes the pattern, rules out other common medical causes of these symptoms, and prescribes an effective antidepressant medication.

• •

Ann, a 40-year-old schoolteacher and single mom, usually lights up the room, but today she arrives for her annual physical looking flat. Dr. Abernathy notes the change, so when running through a checklist of symptoms pauses emphatically on the question about her "spirits." Ann hesitates, then admits that she has been feeling "run down and stressed out" for over a month. Questioned further, she confesses that she has fallen way behind on grading and lesson plans and is beginning to worry she might never get through them. She has all but stopped lecturing to her fifth graders. Yesterday she retreated to the back of the room so she could put her head down while the students watched educational videos and scribbled in workbooks.

Dr. Abernathy asks about her energy level. Ann sighs and says that she goes straight to bed when she gets home from work. She wishes she could sleep, but she cannot. Instead, she lies awake for hours staring at the ceiling, too tired and apathetic to move. Fortunately her teenage daughter can feed herself and deal with her own homework. After a long struggle to fall asleep, Ann is usually up again at 4:00 a.m., unable to find another moment of rest. Ann has no appetite, and according to the clinic scale has lost ten pounds from her already slight frame since her last visit one year ago. (1) During her long hours awake in bed, she wishes she could find distraction in a novel or a movie, but she can't focus on anything long enough to get into the plot or care what happens. (2) Although the thought of suicide fills her with dread, she finds herself fantasizing about disappearing, simply not existing, and she has started to think that maybe she is such a drain on her family that they would be better off if she were not around. (3)

Ann cannot think of anything going on in her life that could be making her feel so miserable—on a daily basis she finds herself crying over nothing. (4) She has had similar down periods from time to time in the past. Usually she can pin them to some major event, like a death in the family or a stressful work situation, but they pass in a week or two, unlike this one. (5)

Dr. Abernathy asks her about other physical symptoms

and orders a set of basic laboratory studies, including thyroid hormone function, but Ann appears physically well, has regular periods and normal vital signs, and there are no abnormalities on her physical exam. (6) Dr. Abernathy tells her she has a major depressive disorder. Ann is not completely surprised by this diagnosis, as her mother had gone through similar times of depression and was successfully treated with an unknown medication. (7) Dr. Abernathy and Ann review some treatment options. Although counseling is offered as an option, Dr. Abernathy strongly recommends that she go on an antidepressant medication. They consider her specific symptoms—insomnia and diminished appetite especially—and decide on a drug that tends to be sedating and that has a side effect of stimulating the appetite. (8)

Ann starts on the antidepressant and notices right away some improvement in sleep and appetite, though no other marked change in other depressive symptoms in the first few weeks. (9) She checks in with Dr. Abernathy several times in the first few weeks to confirm that she is having no unpleasant side effects and that she is ready to advance to the next dose. After three weeks on the higher dose, Ann begins to notice that she has an easier time fighting the urge to withdraw to bed, and by week four she is digging into the backlog of homework to be graded, spending more time with her daughter in the evening, and tending to some deferred household projects. Still, Ann experiences some lethargy, and she has not yet begun to feel better, just to notice that she has the capacity to do more. Over the next several weeks the mood begins to lift, and by the eighth week, when she checks in with Dr. Abernathy at the clinic, Ann appears once again bright and engaging, neatly groomed, and she happily reports that she feels fully back to normal. (10)

Summary: Textbook Depression

●●●

Basic facts about major depressive disorder

- ▶ A medical illness defined by a set of symptoms that cluster together for two weeks (but usually much longer) and cause significant distress and functional impairment. The symptoms must include low mood and/or a diminished enjoyment or satisfaction in one's usual activities, combined with some combination of:
  - ▷ feelings of guilt or worthlessness
  - ▷ diminished energy
  - ▷ diminished ability to think or concentrate, or indecisiveness
  - ▷ changes in sleep (too much or too little)
  - ▷ changes in appetite (too much or too little)
  - ▷ either a slowing of activity ("psychomotor retardation") or agitation
  - ▷ suicidal thoughts or wishes for death.
- ▶ Major depressive disorder affects between 5 and 20 percent of the population over the course of a lifetime (depending on how the disorder is defined and diagnosed, and what the study population is).
- ▶ Women are about twice as likely as men to have depression (until after menopausal age, when the rates equalize).
- ▶ First episodes tend to occur once individuals reach their twenties, but depression occurring for the first time in the elderly is not uncommon as a complication of medical disorders and grief.
- ▶ Major depressive disorder is associated with higher risk of medical illness. Those with a medical illness tend to have poorer prognoses.

▸ Major depressive disorder is the largest single risk factor for disability worldwide and is the strongest predictor of suicide. Among people who have severe major depressive disorder, the risk of suicide is about one hundred times greater than the rate in the general population.

Basic facts about antidepressant therapy

▸ The effectiveness of antidepressant therapy for severe major depressive disorder has been established consistently for sixty years. Effectiveness for milder forms of depression is not as well established.

▸ Antidepressant medications help in about 60 to 70 percent of cases, and symptoms resolve completely in about half of these. Lingering distress and risk for relapse can limit the benefits of apparently successful treatment, however.

▸ Newer antidepressants account for most of the cost of treating depression, and that cost has risen sharply over the past twenty-five years. While in some cases their side effects, if any, are easier to tolerate, the newer antidepressants work no better or worse than the older (and cheaper) ones.

▸ All currently available drugs classified as antidepressants seem to work by increasing the amount of the neurotransmitters serotonin and/or norepinephrine (and possibly dopamine) in the space between neurons in the brain. But it is not known why this change in neurotransmitters results in an effective antidepressant treatment.

Case Notes

∙∙∙

(1) Based on Ann's symptoms, this is a textbook case of major depressive disorder.

(2) Among the symptoms of depression, one is probably

essential to making a definitive diagnosis: anhedonia, or the inability to be motivated to find pleasure or satisfaction in usual activities. The reason is simple. If the capacity to pursue and enjoy usual activities remained intact, the person would either do them and no longer feel depressed, or work to find opportunities to pursue satisfying activities.

(3) Low self-worth often accompanies major depressive disorder. It is insidious, painful, and at times dangerous, when it convinces a person that he or she is of no value to other people and thus forms a rationale for suicide.

(4) The relationship between stress and major depressive disorder is complicated. Stressful conditions can give rise to major depression, but at the same time, major depression can make situations more stressful—directly, by the painfulness of symptoms, and indirectly, by the constraints depression imposes on adaptive behavior.

(5) This history suggests that in her younger years Ann may have had milder, more manageable episodes of major depressive disorder, consistent with an age at onset that tends to occur in people in their twenties.

(6) There are no blood tests or brain scans that can confirm the diagnosis of major depressive disorder, but there are medical disorders that can cause depressive symptoms before causing noticeable physical symptoms. Many of these illnesses can be picked up on routine history, physical, and screening labs plus a thyroid function study.

(7) Having a close relative with major depressive disorder raises one's own likelihood of having it by a factor of about five. There is ample evidence from studies of families, twins, and adoptees to suggest there is a genetic component to the inherit-

Table 1. Antidepressants available in the United States, 2016

Drug Group	Generic Name	Brand Name
Selective serotonin reuptake inhibitor (SSRI)	Citalopram	Celexa
	Escitalopram	Lexapro
	Fluoxetine	Prozac
	Fluvoxamine	Luvox
	Paroxetine	Paxil
	Sertraline	Zoloft
Serotonin-norepinephrine reuptake inhibitor (SNRI)	Venlafaxine	Effexor
	Duloxetine	Cymbalta
	Milnacipran	Savella
	Levomilnacipran	Fetzima
Tricyclic antidepressants (TCAs)	Trimipramine	Surmontil
	Desipramine	Norpramin
	Nortriptyline	Pamelor
	Amoxapine	Asendin
	Maprotiline	Ludiomil
	Amitriptyline	Elavil
	Doxepin	Sinequan
	Imipramine	Tofranil
	Protriptyline	Vivactil
	Clomipramine	Anafranil
Monoamine oxidase inhibitors (MAOIs)	Phenelzine	Nardil
	Selegiline (patch)	Emsam
	Isocarboxacid	Marplan
	Tranylcypromine	Parnate
Other	Mirtazapine	Remeron
	Bupropion	Wellbutrin
	Nefazodone	Serzone
	Trazodone	Desyrel
	Vilazodone	Viibryd
	Vortioxetine	Brintellix

Note: This list includes only medications commonly classified as antidepressants and is not a list of every medication that might be effective for treating major depressive disorder.

ability of depression, but no specific genes have been identified as the cause of mood disorders.

(8) Clinical trials suggest that all antidepressants are equally likely to benefit someone who has major depressive disorder. Typically there is a two out of three chance of significant symptom improvement and one out of three chance of full remission of symptoms for a person taking any appropriate drug. Table 1 lists antidepressants available in the United States in 2016.

(9) As a rule, people will begin to experience the side effects of medication before they experience the benefits. The lag time between the initial drug effects and the alleviation of major depression can be considered evidence against the popular idea that major depression is literally a "chemical imbalance." The early effects demonstrate that the neurotransmitter levels change quickly; the relief of depression must occur through some other, secondary effects of altering neurotransmitter levels.

(10) Symptoms generally improve, at different rates, over a course of six to eight weeks. Sleep and appetite tend to improve first, followed by an apparent increased interest in other people and events (perhaps not noticed by the person who has depression), increased energy, and finally an improvement in the person's own sense of being depressed.

B O B

Treatment Ambivalence

OVERVIEW: Bob is a college student whose progress has been interrupted by major depressive disorder. Although he makes a visit to the campus health center and receives treatment early in the course of his illness, he responds poorly to antidepressants, largely because he does not take the medications regularly. When his family physician finally persuades Bob to stick with the treatment as prescribed, he does much better.

Early in winter break, Bob rushes into the campus health clinic forty minutes late for his eleven o'clock appointment, looking rumpled and unkempt, explaining he overslept and came over as fast as he could. Bob is 21 years old, a junior, and this is the first time he has visited the clinic. Aside from his dishevelment, a worried expression, and some restlessness in the waiting room, he appears well. Fortunately there has been a cancellation, so Dr. Beasly is able to squeeze him in. Bob jumps right to the problem: his parents are upset about his fall semester grades, which included no As, only one B, some Cs, a D, and an Incomplete. Bob grumbles that he really thought he could handle this situation on his own, but his parents wouldn't pay for the next semester unless he got checked out. (1)

Dr. Beasly quickly establishes that Bob's physical health seems unchanged, but that Bob has not been himself the past few months. Previously a conscientious student, he has recently missed a lot of classes, often oversleeping through morning lectures even though he gets to bed well before midnight. It seems like it takes him twice as long to read a page in a textbook, and, worse, Bob finds that he just doesn't care about classes or anything else as much as he used to. He hasn't dated in months and has avoided friends by screening his phone calls and not answering texts, because he would rather go home, "chill," watch videos, and go to bed. He also stopped working out and has gained a paunch in the past few months.

"My folks think I'm drinking too much or using drugs or something," Bob explains. He allows that he does smoke a joint and have a beer or two every evening, but he believes this is no more than what anyone else he knows does. He admits the frequency of use is higher than in his earlier college years, when he confined his drinking to weekends and rarely used pot. (2) He explains that it's the only way he can relax.

"What did you do to relax before?" asks Dr. Beasly.

"Oh, I dunno...play video games, toss the Frisbee, hang out with friends, work at the soup kitchen..."

"And none of these activities is relaxing anymore?"

"No, they all seem kinda pointless." Bob pauses a moment to reflect. "What do you think? Am I becoming an addict?"

Dr. Beasly says, "The pot and the drinking aren't helping, but there's a reason you're using more of it than you used to. As you said, you're not getting any pleasure from the things that usually make you feel good. The reason for that, on top of the changes in your sleep and your weight and energy and ability to do mental work, is that you have depression—not just a bad mood, but clinical depression."

Bob dismisses the idea that he could have a mental illness. He says he wants to just "tough it out," but he is ultimately persuaded to accept a prescription for an antidepressant. Typing away at the electronic medical record on the computer, Dr. Beasly misses Bob's rolling eyes while advising Bob that some studies have found that people may experience an increase in urges for suicide and self-harm when starting on an antidepressant. Bob should return in a week just to be on the safe side. (3)

At the one-week check-in, Bob is no better. When pressed, he admits he has not started the drug. He had gone to fill the prescription but found that there was no generic version and a high co-pay on his parents' insurance plan, so he blew it off. (4) Dr. Beasly offers him a different agent, one that is approved for coverage by the insurance company, and admonishes him to call next time if he has any problems. Bob fills the prescription and at first struggles to remember to take it, but he is too embarrassed to confess his forgetfulness when he calls to check in, still no better, the following week. Unaware of Bob's spotty medication habits, Dr. Beasly advises him to double the dose, which he does, and he begins to take the medication regularly. As the second week progresses, Bob notices he is becoming more easily frustrated and snappish, and has the urge to break things or knock over people who get in his way. He calls and reports these feelings to Dr. Beasly, who advises him to back down on the dose and to advance it more gradually. (5) But this too brings on irritability, and out of frustration Bob once again discontinues the medication and treatment, seeing them as a waste of time.

A few weeks later, Bob's mother calls the campus clinic to try to understand why Bob remains depressed. Dr. Beasly's nurse offers to find out and so reaches out to Bob to ask why he hasn't followed up. Bob again has to admit that he stopped the drug and that his mood is "still down." Dr. Beasly prescribes another antidepressant and advises him to advance very gradually on the dose. Still skeptical, Bob agrees to try, and within one month he is on a dose in the low therapeutic range. Although he doesn't feel any better, he notes he is having an easier time getting to class and keeping up with the reading, and he has begun to have a glimmer of interest in sex once again. He is too embarrassed to mention, however, that it seems to be taking him a long time to climax when he masturbates, and believes it might not be from the drug but from being out of practice. Another week goes by with no further improvement in either his mood or his sexual performance, so out of frustration he once again stops his medication. (6)

By this time the semester is well underway. Still struggling with his inertia, Bob is able to just barely keep his head above water and to finish the year with a B average and no further contact with the campus health clinic. But he has made no plans for the summer and returns to his parents' home and his old bedroom, from which he rarely emerges. His parents take him to their family doctor, Dr. Boyd.

Bob describes his symptoms and explains his frustration with the antidepressant treatment. Dr. Boyd acknowledges that his side effects were fairly common but assures him that they can be avoided, and explains that the medications must be taken daily at the full dose for many weeks before he can expect satisfactory improvement. Dr. Boyd also insists that Bob should take a break from alcohol and marijuana, in order to give the medications an optimal chance to work. Bob remarks that his college doctor had not made these points clear before. Dr. Boyd prescribes a different antidepressant, one with low potential for sexual side effects and that is somewhat activating, to help with Bob's inertia, but advances it gradually to avoid the irritability Bob had experienced before. (7)

With Dr. Boyd's guidance, Bob is able to stick with the medication all summer and approaches his senior year with an enthusiasm he hadn't felt in several years. He thrives in class and secures a place in a graduate program. The following summer, after graduation, he asks if he could stop the medication. He has no particular reason for wanting to do so, other than to be free of the burden of having to remember to take medications. Dr. Boyd agrees, gingerly, and Bob gradually withdraws the medication over the next month, checking in weekly with Dr. Boyd. (8) But as Bob drops below the halfway point on the dose, he notices some of the symptoms returning. So he continues the drug at half the dose he took previously, and remains on that dose during his transition to graduate school.

Summary: Treatment Ambivalence

▸ Many patients do not take medications exactly as prescribed. This is particularly a problem when the medications have no immediate positive effect but instead require faithful adherence over many weeks before an effect can be expected.

▶ Treating depression involves more than just writing a prescription; many patients must be educated and enlisted as active participants in their treatment.

▶ The prudent clinician does close follow-up on a patient who is newly starting an antidepressant, especially a younger person who may become agitated when initiating medication treatment.

▶ Recommendations for continuation of treatment vary from a minimum of three months after recovery to indefinitely. When in doubt, the medication may be tapered gradually, to reveal whether the patient will continue to benefit from the drug or whether it can be discontinued without consequence.

Case Notes
....

(1) An abnormal mood state can be, and often is, confused with the natural emotional volatility of youth. The best indicator of a major depressive disorder may be a change in functioning, rather than a change in mood. Examples of changes in functioning are declining grades, waning interest in hobbies, dropping out of school activities that used to be compelling, or abrupt changes in friends.

(2) Occasional drug use is common among younger people, but new onset of habitual drug use is a common complication of major depressive disorder. Drugs of abuse along with other highly stimulating activities like self-cutting, shoplifting, and bulimia bypass the normal mechanisms by which appetites

and life goals are rewarded and satisfied, and may seem to the depressed person to be the only way to feel better.

(3) Reports of new suicidal thinking among adolescents starting antidepressant medications have prompted the requirement that antidepressants carry a warning label. But there is no evidence of an increased rate of completed suicide arising from antidepressant use. Although there is good reason to believe that the risk of suicide and self-harm from *not* treating depression far outweighs the risk of this purported side effect, the language of the warning advises only that the physician who prescribes the medications should closely observe such patients (say, with weekly contact or visits). This is sound advice.

(4) Not taking medications on the prescribed schedule or at the prescribed dosage in many circumstances is more the rule than the exception.

(5) Agitation can be an early side effect of an antidepressant and is particularly concerning in young people, who have poorer impulse control than they are likely to develop once fully matured.

(6) Sexual side effects are common with some antidepressants and can be unpleasant to experience and embarrassing to discuss.

(7) The best all-around remedy for poor treatment adherence is for physician and patient to work together to establish goals and agree on the means to achieve them. The physician's role may often be to inspire the patient to collaborate. In contrast, ordering the patient to cooperate tends to lead to therapeutic failure.

(8) Duration of antidepressant treatment depends on many factors, including the severity of the illness, the difficulty

of achieving a therapeutic response, and the frequency of recurrences. Stopping medications is a time for *increased*, not decreased, surveillance by the physician, at least until it can be established that the drug is not necessary.

CARLA

Underdosing

....

OVERVIEW: Carla's anxiety—a function both of her personality
and of her state of major depressive disorder—manifests in
exaggerated concerns about her physical health and an inability
to tolerate any medication side effects, real or imagined. Her
primary care provider, unable to get her onto an adequate antidepressant regimen, refers her to a psychiatrist, who persuades
her to advance very slowly onto a new antidepressant, until she
finally responds.

....

It is Carla's first visit to a psychiatrist, and she is visibly anxious.
She is a tired-appearing 55-year-old widow and lifelong home-
maker, but her eye contact with the psychiatrist, Dr. Clark, can

best be described as a glare, as if she were challenging, *I dare you to try to help me.*

"I think I'm beyond help," she says, and then she names the three antidepressant medications her primary care physician, Dr. Cohen, has prescribed for her since she began treatment for her depressive episode three months ago. "None of them work," she reports. "I've tried everything and I'm still down."

Dr. Clark takes note of the list and asks Carla to describe her depression. "I've never really felt sad," she says, "which may be one reason it took me a long time to realize there was something wrong with me, that I was not just being overstressed by life." Dr. Clark asks her when she last felt well, and how she came to the conclusion there was something wrong. At first she names the exact date five years ago that her husband died suddenly, of a cerebral aneurysm, and then she adds that all things considered she probably coped with his death about as well as could be expected. Although saddened and shocked by the loss, she was able to take comfort in her friends and church activities. (1)

On second thought, Carla now recalls, things started to go downhill about six months ago, while she was on a country retreat with a group of friends, playing cards. Out of nowhere she felt flushed, sweaty, shaky, her heart practically beating out of her chest, and she was terrified she might be having a heart attack. Because they were miles from town, by the time an ambulance arrived she was feeling physically okay, albeit a little drained, and declined to go to the hospital. A quick Internet search convinced her that she had experienced a panic attack.

Carla had no more panic attacks in the weeks that followed, but she continued to feel uneasy. At first her uneasiness was confined to the morning, but it spread to a general sense of dread and fear that she carried with her all the time, which was a dramatic change from her usual self-assured independence. She began to lie awake nights, pondering the consequences if the stock market were to crash and struggling with the persistent thought that she could become homeless within a matter of weeks. (2)

As weeks wore on, she felt a growing sense of fatigue, lost interest in food, and experienced "muzzy-headedness" that made it too difficult to follow the plots of the mystery novels she usually enjoyed. She also noticed that she was visiting the bathroom more often and more urgently, and she worried that she had ingested a parasite. She began to wake up with a headache nearly every day. On one occasion she experienced sharp pains around her throat and was convinced she could feel enlarged and tender lymph nodes, until Dr. Cohen reassured her there was nothing to worry about, and that Carla's constant pressing on her neck was what made it sore. (3)

It was while evaluating Carla during an office visit about her neck that Dr. Cohen began to suspect that Carla had major depressive disorder. (4) Prescribing a popular selective serotonin reuptake inhibitor (SSRI), Dr. Cohen explained to Carla that she might experience headache or nausea when first taking it, but that these symptoms would likely clear up within a few weeks. (5)

Carla began the SSRI the next morning. The same evening, Dr. Cohen received an urgent page concerning Carla, who was having a "bad reaction" to the medication. When Dr. Cohen called Carla back, Carla told Dr. Cohen that she had a headache, upset stomach, and an uncontrollable urge to keep moving, with shaking limbs, pacing, wringing hands, and so on. She was certain she would be too wound up to be able to sleep that night. Unable to see her or to prescribe a stronger anxiety pill by phone, Dr. Cohen advised her to take an over-the-counter sleep aid and to come in the next day.

The next day Dr. Cohen learned that Carla had managed to get through the night with her usual six hours of broken sleep. Despite suspicions that the "bad reaction" was probably psychosomatic and related to her depression, Carla could not be convinced to continue taking the antidepressant. So she was prescribed an alternative antidepressant (6) known for having a more sedating quality to it, and she promised to give the new drug a try. The only immediate effect she noticed after starting it was a ravenous hunger. After four days, Carla contacted Dr. Cohen to report that she could take the drug no longer, as a friend had told her (and the Internet had confirmed) that the drug caused weight gain. Dr. Cohen reflected to her that she was, if anything, underweight at the moment and could probably stand to add a few pounds, but Carla was stuck on the idea of getting "fat" and wouldn't consider staying with the medication.

Mildly flummoxed, Dr. Cohen selected another, less familiar antidepressant; although side effects in general were no better with this drug, it was not associated with weight gain and had the advantage of being available in small increments, so the dose could be advanced gradually. (7) Carla was told to start with the smallest dose, and to take only half a pill for the first week, and then to advance to a full pill by the following week. At the end of two weeks they would meet again to see where they should go. At the end of the first week, however, Carla called to report that she was feeling "racy" on the new medication, with a daily headache and feelings of gastric bloating, and she said she did not want to increase the dose. She agreed to give the half pill another week and to come in for her planned appointment the following week.

When she again visited Dr. Cohen, she was still having the racy feelings, headache, and bloating, though the symptoms were a bit milder. Carla would only agree to stay on the half pill, despite Dr. Cohen's warning that she would probably not experience any antidepressant effect until she was taking a considerably higher dose of the drug. After two more weeks on the half pill, the headache and bloating had subsided enough that Carla was willing to take a whole pill. She remained just as miserable from both the depression and the physical symptoms for another month before she could be persuaded to add a second pill, but with this increase the symptoms became intolerable. She tried to stop the drug entirely but then experienced many of the discontinuation symptoms she had read about on the Internet, so she stayed with the one-pill dose until she could see Dr. Cohen again. At this point Dr. Cohen admitted to being out of new ideas and referred Carla to a psychiatrist, Dr. Clark (8).

Today, at the time of her first visit to Dr. Clark, Carla is still taking the miniscule dose of one pill daily from the previous prescription started six weeks ago, and she remains hesitant to increase the dose again. Her symptoms of anxiety and depression are, if anything, worse than when she first sought help from Dr. Cohen; she can no longer tolerate being around her friends, as she has become intensely worried about having an embarrassing bout of diarrhea, or feeling too overwhelmed by headache to complete a game of cards.

Dr. Clark proposes a new tack in the form of an old drug. Nortriptyline is the only antidepressant with a well-established, measurable therapeutic window—a range of blood levels the drug works optimally within as demonstrated in controlled studies. Although the side effects tend to be more noticeable than those of the newer agents, nortriptyline can be prescribed in extremely small increments to allow for precise dosing. Dr. Clark points out, "At least we'll know whether your brain is seeing enough of the drug to explain your 'side effects' or to get you better."

Carla starts on the smallest possible dose—about one-tenth of the usual therapeutic dose—and, aside from the typical side effect of dry mouth, her headache, bloating, and restlessness are no worse than before. When she balks at increasing the dose further, Dr. Clark has a frank talk with her about the need to commit herself to a course of antidepressants, emphasizing that it is not at all clear her symptoms are side effects; rather, they are probably benign sensations amplified to the level of severe discomfort by her state of depression. (9) Dr. Clark prescribes an antianxiety agent (just for the short term) to try to facilitate her adjustment to the medication.

Seeing no alternative, and soothed a bit by the antianxiety agent, Carla agrees to advance the dose. On a dose about half of the usual therapeutic dose, Dr. Clark orders a blood test to check the amount of drug in her system and is surprised to see that Carla has already crossed into the low end of the therapeutic range. (10) After three weeks on this dose, Carla admits that her sleep has definitely improved and she is having an easier time getting her day started. She is even beginning to look forward to getting out of the house to do things. She is planning to meet a friend next week, one on one, and although she is apprehensive, she also is hopeful that it will be a good outing. By week eight, Carla is still only partially better, and her blood level is still in the low end of the therapeutic range, so with some trepidation they increase the nortriptyline dose again, slightly, bringing her to about two-thirds of the usual therapeutic dosage, but when her blood level is measured it brings her to the middle of the therapeutic range. (11) Carla tolerates the increase without a problem and continues to improve toward full recovery over the subsequent month.

Summary: Underdosing

- ▶ Many people with certain forms of depression—particularly anxious depression—mistakenly categorize physical symptoms of the disorder as drug side effects.
- ▶ Impediments to treatment caused by anxious symptoms or side effects, or anxious symptoms appearing as side effects, can be overcome if the clinician provides additional psychological support to the patient.
- ▶ Variability among individuals in what dose is effective and how they respond to the medication is largely a function of how rapidly the body eliminates the drug. A few psychiatric drugs are excreted through the kidneys, so elimination is determined by how efficiently the kidneys filter the bloodstream. Most antidepressants are eliminated by liver enzymes, which break down, or metabolize, the chemical components of drugs. Genetic variation in these enzymes leads to variability in the efficiency of drug metabolism in different individuals.
- ▶ Genetic research has led recently to the development of commercially available tests that can predict how efficiently an individual might process a given drug. The tests cannot say how effective a given drug might be for an individual, but rather whether an individual is likely to tolerate or have

a therapeutic response to the standard dose of the specific drug.

► Again, therapeutic collaboration is the key to successful treatment.

Case Notes
••

(1) After losing her husband, Carla was in a state of bereavement, not major depressive disorder. Normal bereavement can be differentiated from a grief-triggered major depressive episode by the ability to carry on with normal life functions and to experience pleasure when it is available. Bereavement can lead to major depressive disorder, however. If the loss of a loved one leads to functional impairment and the loss of motivation to pursue normal, pleasurable activities, then antidepressant treatment may be indicated.

(2) Anxiety is a common and agonizing symptom of depression in many people. A persistently anxious mood or bouts of intense anxiety may emerge as a symptom of major depression or as a complication of life stress secondary to depression, or they may reflect an exaggerated expression of personality vulnerabilities.

(3) Anxiety and depression fuel psychosomatic symptoms. With or without anxiety, a person with all of the symptoms of major depressive disorder may be more concerned with and may complain more about physical symptoms than about having a low mood, because in some cultures a low mood is thought to reflect weakness.

(4) Primary care providers are very much on the front lines of treatment for major depressive disorder, and they treat the majority of patients. But most of them become comfortable

with prescribing only a few of the available antidepressant medications.

(5) SSRIs are most often the first antidepressants prescribed. Starting with fluoxetine (Prozac) in the late 1980s, a variety of these generally effective, well-tolerated, easy-to-use, safe medications have emerged.

(6) When drugs from one class do not work, it is worth trying drugs from a different class. At this time there is no reliable way to establish in advance which patients will do best on which classes of antidepressants, so trial and error informed by knowledge about past trials is as good a method as any.

(7) For people who are so sensitive to side effects that they cannot tolerate a therapeutic dose, it may be helpful to start low and go slow.

(8) When the primary care provider has made a few unsuccessful attempts at treatment, or when the severity of the illness is such that more intensive pharmacologic and psychotherapeutic intervention is needed, then the primary care provider may refer the patient to a psychiatrist.

(9) Medications can, of course, induce unpleasant side effects in the form of physical symptoms, but common symptoms like headache and gastric upset occur frequently with or without medications. In experimental drug trials, even participants receiving placebo report side effects, so there is some justification in doubting that every reported symptom is a true side effect of the medication.

(10) Many factors may determine how much of the drug enters the system and reaches the brain. Variations in these factors can work against effective treatment, in either direction: if a given dose of a drug leads to a blood level lower than expected,

then the brain never sees a sufficient amount of it to generate a response. If the level is higher than expected, then side effects may arise so early in treatment that a patient will not tolerate or take the drug long enough for it to work.

(11) Dr. Clark's success engaging Carla in a therapeutic collaboration, combined with information about the amount of drug in her system, supported the last dosage increase to push her to the middle of the therapeutic range and full recovery.

II : MISDIAGNOSIS

The stories in this section illustrate problems that can occur when antidepressants are prescribed for people who appear superficially to have major depressive disorder, but who on closer examination have something else that resembles it.

DARIUS

Demoralization

• •

OVERVIEW: Darius has already gone through several psychiatrists who have been unable to find the right antidepressant
medication for his depressive symptoms. A thorough history
confirms that Darius feels depressed and has several associated
depressive symptoms, but it also suggests that he may not have
a major depressive disorder. The persistence, pervasiveness, and
severity of his symptoms fall short of the diagnostic standard
for major depression. He may actually be demoralized—under-
standably so—about a series of life setbacks. Rather than using
yet another antidepressant, Darius tries psychotherapy, which
helps him to take some positive steps toward making his life
more satisfying.

• •

Darius, a 38-year-old divorced former small business owner (and current warehouse manager), is now seeing his third psychiatrist. "I thought I was having a midlife crisis," he begins, "but they told me I have depression. Problem is, nothing helps. The other docs ran out of ideas. Maybe you can think of something fresh."

Looking at Darius, one might not think he's depressed. He is freshly shaved, sporting a neat, short haircut, and he is wearing worn but clean jeans, sneakers, and blank t-shirt. Although somewhat glum, he is easily engaged to tell his story. He speaks freely and fluidly, with animated gestures. "They tried this, they tried that, they tried something else, they tried combinations, but nothing worked. Do you think maybe I need shock treatments?"

Brushing off the last question with a quick "probably not," (1) the psychiatrist, Dr. Dennis, gathers the story from Darius and from the previous psychiatrist's records. Darius had initially been referred for psychiatric treatment five years ago, after he had made a "suicidal statement" to the marriage counselor he and his wife had been seeing. As Darius recalls it now, what he actually said, in a moment of intense frustration, was "Maybe I should just drive off a cliff or something." He said it in anger, without any intention of taking suicidal action, but he went along with the psychiatric referral anyway, because he thought it might help save the marriage. But the marriage was doomed; he had suspected when they went into counseling that his now ex-wife was only having a "fling," and he was hoping she would just admit it so they could put it behind them and get on with life. What he learned, however, was that his wife was having an affair with his business partner, and that it was serious.

This revelation was the tipping point for Darius. "I was
a happy-go-lucky kind of guy. I loved my wife, my kids, my
boat, my business. Life was really good. Then, whoosh, down
the drain." Dr. Dennis asks him to elaborate on that period of
stress. Darius recalls that there was a yearlong period when
he was talking to his lawyer constantly, running up huge legal
bills, fighting his wife for custody of the kids and property, and
fighting his partner for the business. In the end the business
had to be dissolved, and a large chunk of the proceeds went
to pay legal bills. He was happy to have custody of the kids on
weekends and holidays, for two weeks in the summer, and to
have been able to keep his boat despite the ruinous property
settlement. (2)

Darius took the warehouse job just to stay afloat, intend-
ing to start up a new business within the year, but four years
have gone by and he's still there. For a while after the divorce
he avoided relationships, and then had a series of brief and
unsatisfying forays into online dating, but now he thinks it's
not worth the trouble. His sleep is "totally effed up." The job
has him working on a rotating shift basis, so every third week
he's there all night, and by the time he's able to put together
six hours of solid sleep during the day, it is time to work the
day shift again. On days when he's not working and his kids
are not around, he can sleep most of the day. His weight has
steadily risen, and he is thirty pounds heavier than four years
ago, partly, he thinks, attributable to medication side effects,
but mostly from poor eating habits. During the workweek when
he's not sleeping, Darius doesn't have enough energy to do
anything else, so he tends to just hole up in his room watching
his chronically disappointing local sports teams. (3)

The only thing he has consistently looked forward to is the

time he spends with his kids. They were both young at the time of the divorce—7 and 9 years old—and there was little need to plan anything for their weekends together, as they were content spending time on the boat, going to a ballgame or to the movies, or playing miniature golf. Now that they have hit puberty, however, it seems harder and harder to rouse their enthusiasm for these spontaneous activities. He's about ready to give up trying to think of fun things for them to do. He fantasizes about going out more on his boat, but with the kids losing interest and his free time taken up with them, he finds he has even less time to enjoy boating. (4)

"So, doc, I'm in a rut. I'm unhappy, I'm tired all the time, I never get enough sleep, I've gotten fat eating junk food, and it seems like things are just getting worse. I'm not having any fun at all, and I'm too lazy to do anything about it. I guess I'm depressed." The first psychiatrist he saw came to the same conclusion and started him on an SSRI antidepressant. (5) "No side effects, but no good effects" was the verdict.

When the standard dose had no effect, positive or negative, the psychiatrist pushed the dose higher and higher. "It was weird. At the max dose I didn't feel down anymore, but I didn't feel normal either. I just didn't care. I'm usually kind of a neatnik, but I stopped vacuuming, doing laundry, washing dishes, everything. When my kids would come over, we'd spend the day watching cartoons. After a couple of weeks of that, even the kids started to complain about not doing anything, so I mentioned it to the doc." The psychiatrist thought he was experiencing an SSRI-induced apathy syndrome (6) and switched him to a different drug, one that was not an SSRI. The apathy cleared but Darius still felt down, so he decided he needed a new psychiatrist. His new doctor started yet another antidepressant, which only made him feel a little jittery and "wired." Darius had taken each of the antidepressants for two months or more at standard therapeutic doses (or higher) and essentially had no benefit. The second psychiatrist, daunted by Darius's failure with the first psychiatrist and with the new medication, referred him to Dr. Dennis, who is widely acknowledged by peers as a mood disorder expert.

Dr. Dennis reviews Darius's symptoms: low mood, low energy, disrupted sleep, weight gain, low self-esteem (calling himself "lazy"), feelings of hopelessness, loss of interest in sex. "You certainly feel depressed," Dr. Dennis adds, "but I suspect you may not have major depressive disorder, for two reasons. First, although you have many of the symptoms of depression, strictly speaking they probably haven't been severe enough to count toward a diagnosis of major depression—you've still been able to work and entertain your kids, and you haven't been suicidal. Second, and I think most importantly, you are still able to enjoy things when you have the opportunity. People with major depression can't enjoy things even when they have the chance." (7)

"Yeah, I guess that makes sense," says Darius. "I took the kids to a water park last month—they were begging me to go—and I probably had more fun than they did. I forgot about that. So you're saying there's a difference between feeling depressed and having major depressive disorder. Does that make a difference in how well antidepressants work?"

"Definitely. Depressed mood is a normal response to severe adversity. Major depression arises from a disruption of normal brain activity. For depressed mood, a change of circumstances or a better adaptation to circumstances is required. For major depression, antidepressant medication works better. Interestingly, in antidepressant drug trials, the evidence is that they work much better for people with severe major depression than for people like you, who have milder symptoms and impairment."

"Then why did those other psychiatrists keep giving me antidepressant pills when I didn't really have major depression?" Darius asks. (8)

"If I had been the first psychiatrist to see you, I probably would have recommended an antidepressant, too, just in case I was missing something—say, if you really did have major depression but were describing only mild symptoms because it was early in the course of the illness, or because you were compensating well. In that case, the risk from taking medication was low and the potential benefit would have been high. In retrospect, it would have made sense to put more emphasis on getting you into some psychotherapy right from the start." Dr. Dennis thinks cognitive-behavioral therapy (CBT) might be particularly helpful because of the cognitive distortions observed in Darius's account, such as seeing no point in planning weekend outings because "the kids are going to hate it no matter what I do." (9) Dr. Dennis also discusses sleep hygiene with him and recommends melatonin to ease the transitions in shiftwork. Taking note of Darius's weight gain, Dr. Dennis considers the possibility of obstructive sleep apnea as a contributing factor to his sleeplessness and fatigue. A sleep study rules out sleep apnea as a factor in his poor sleep, but in subsequent weeks Darius adopts a habit of daily walks and finds that it brightens his outlook and helps regulate sleep.

Over the course of twelve sessions, Darius is able to push past some of the obstacles to getting back into a satisfying career, and he is excited for the first time in a long time about a woman he had met in the household cleaning products aisle of the supermarket. She was impressed with his knowledge of nonabrasive cleansers and would be meeting him for a second date next week. He has also made it a point to talk with his kids about what kinds of activities they would enjoy doing with him on weekends, including just hanging out sometimes, and so he is having better luck planning things they all enjoy.

Summary: Demoralization

▸ Because many of the symptoms of depression are not exclusively symptoms of depression, there is no vivid distinction between major depressive disorder, which few would dispute is a serious mental illness, and demoralization, which is not an illness but is an understandable reaction that can occur to almost anyone under adverse circumstances.

▸ To further complicate matters, major depressive disorder is itself extremely demoralizing. If a person, before experiencing major depression, has a set of strategies to cope with bad times by engaging in rewarding activities, then the core deficit of major depression—the loss of a capacity to feel reward or satisfaction—takes away the potential for those strategies to succeed, leaving the person with no effective way to cope. This sense of helplessness is the essence of demoralization.

▸ For many people, antidepressant medications are more accessible (affordable, available, reachable, schedulable)

Table 2. Major depression symptoms versus demoralization and bereavement

Symptom	Major Depressive Disorder	Demoralization	Bereavement
Low mood	Usually yes	Yes	Yes
Low self-attitude	Yes	Somewhat	Usually no
Insomnia	Yes	Maybe	Maybe
Low appetite	Yes	No	No
Unable to enjoy things	Yes	No	No
Unable to find things to enjoy	Maybe	Yes	Maybe
Suicidal	Often	Infrequent	No
Triggered by life events	Sometimes	Always	Always

than psychotherapy, so for this reason, as well as because of the uncertain boundary between major depression and demoralization, some demoralized people are being treated with antidepressants from which they are unlikely to benefit.

▶ Not every person with major depression requires psychotherapy to achieve recovery, but any person who has demoralization—that sense of being stuck in a rut with no way out—probably can benefit from some form of psychotherapy, whether or not he or she has major depression.

Case Notes

(1) Electroconvulsive therapy (ECT, or "shock treatments") is the single most effective form of treatment for major depressive disorder, and it is often suggested when someone who has depression does not respond to several antidepressants. But ECT is not ideal for someone who is currently not in acute danger and is able to function adequately. It essentially requires patients to surrender any ongoing responsibility for the

duration of the treatment, because the potential for cognitive impairment, although transient, precludes driving, making important decisions, or engaging in normal, reciprocal social relationships.

(2) The fact that major life stressors may precede a depressive episode has no bearing either way on the diagnosis. Psychiatrists used to differentiate "endogenous" depressions (internally generated) from "reactive" depressions, but there is no difference between them in the treatment response or prognosis.

(3) Other major depression-associated symptoms—in this case sleep disruption, weight gain, and low energy—generally increase the likelihood that someone with a low mood has major depressive disorder. In Darius's case, these symptoms might have other explanations: sleep disruption and fatigue from an erratic work schedule, unhealthy diet, and the like.

(4) Darius can still find things to be happy about, like his boat and the custody arrangements. The key to questioning the diagnosis of major depression in this case is that Darius does not lack the capacity to enjoy himself; rather, he is finding it increasingly difficult to find the opportunity to do so.

(5) Even with the diagnosis of major depression in doubt, the first psychiatrist did not necessarily do the wrong thing by prescribing an antidepressant. For most people, antidepressants are safe and easily tolerated. Based on Darius's symptoms, one could not say with 100 percent certainty that he does *not* have major depressive disorder, so there is little risk—and possibly great benefit—from at least giving an antidepressant a try. As Dr. Dennis will point out later in the session, the problem was in relying exclusively on medications and overlooking psychotherapy.

(6) At high and sometimes at middling doses of SSRIs, a certain percentage of people may experience a state of apathy that is easily confused with depression. But while the person loses the fear normally associated with failing obligations, the capacity for satisfaction and reward remains intact, so this apathy is not a symptom of depression. Such a state of apathy is a good indication of a need to back down on the dose of the SSRI or to eliminate the SSRI.

(7) Dr. Dennis doesn't use the word, and it is not included in the official diagnostic manual for psychiatry, the *Diagnostic and Statistical Manual of Mental Disorders (DSM)*, but perhaps the best descriptive term for Darius's condition is "demoralization." A person in a demoralized state is chronically dissatisfied with life and is unable to perceive any way to improve the situation. It is similar to the *DSM* diagnosis of "adjustment disorder," although the diagnosis of demoralization is more flexible, because demoralization can arise from an internal psychological distress, such as an existential crisis or loss of faith, whereas an adjustment disorder diagnosis requires an inciting event.

(8) Confusion between demoralization and major depressive disorder is likely responsible for much of the controversy in the field about the effectiveness of antidepressant medications. Antidepressants work well for major depression but poorly for demoralization. When there is doubt about the diagnosis, unsuccessful treatment is a result of relying exclusively on antidepressants for treatment when the patient may not have major depressive disorder.

(9) CBT addresses habits of thought that are colored gray by the demoralized state. Starting with the assumption that these

negative expectations inhibit the person from taking the kinds of personal and social risks that are necessary to achieve satisfaction with life, the process of CBT extinguishes the inhibiting effects of these thoughts by highlighting their irrationality.

EVELYN

Bipolar Depression

....

OVERVIEW: Evelyn has had severe major depressions and extremely good, but short-lived, results from antidepressants. During her first visit with a psychiatrist, additional information emerges that suggests these blips in her mood are hypomanic episodes (mild mania), that Evelyn has a bipolar disorder, and that antidepressants may be making her depressions worse. She goes on lithium along with an antidepressant, but she doesn't have a stable recovery until she eliminates the antidepressant.

....

"My antidepressant pooped out. Again. That's why I'm here." Evelyn, a 28-year-old divorced systems analyst, sighs heavily. This is her first visit to the psychiatrist, Dr. Engel, referred by her nurse practitioner (NP) for expert advice. The NP's note

49

richly documents Evelyn's symptoms and treatment trials, as well as her personal history, which Dr. Engel reviews with Evelyn.

Evelyn is the youngest of three daughters of a wayward alcoholic "inventor" and his long-suffering wife. Home life was erratic because Evelyn's father sometimes disappeared for months at a time, leaving the wife and kids to fend for themselves (or turn to Evelyn's grandparents for support); other times he seemed to spend all his time in bed. Growing up in a conservative, midwestern community, Evelyn was sheltered by a strong religious upbringing. She had always liked school and had done well academically and socially, despite some awkwardness when she realized she was more attracted to some of the girls she hung out with than to the boys who kept asking her out. She wound up marrying one of those boys during a hiatus from college, on impulse, in Vegas, when she was taking a semester off for a road trip around the country. The marriage lasted about three weeks; they ended it before she had crossed back east over the Rockies.

She was hired right out of college to work in the IT department of a large local company, and she thrived there for a few years. But after earning a promotion and fostering a reputation as a reliable team player, Evelyn got embroiled in some nasty office politics, became increasingly irritable and disengaged, and in a fit of rage told off the CEO. She was promptly fired. There was a recession at the time, so she took the first job she could get, as a waitress, and was holding her own for a few months until she had a "breakdown"—several months during which she cried daily for no reason, lost all motivation for work, slept twelve or more hours a day, and stayed in bed playing computer games most of the rest of the time. She was too tired even to shower very often, subsisting on ice cream and snack chips. Once she reached the point when she lacked enough money in her savings to pay the rent and found herself thinking she might as well just kill herself, Evelyn finally reached out for help to the only health professional she knew: her gynecologist. (1)

The gynecologist put her on an SSRI, and within a few days Evelyn was feeling much, much better. "Not just better from my funk, but better than I had *ever* felt." She promptly talked her sister into lending her rent and grocery money, cleaned up the squalor that had grown around her while she lay in bed, filled her fridge and cupboards, bought a stylish new job-hunting outfit on credit, and within a week landed another job in the IT field. When she had been on the antidepressant for an entire month, she "forgot" to take it for a few days and still felt great, so she left the pill bottle to age past its expiration date in her medicine cabinet.

As for relationships, she had finished college unpartnered, though she had begun to explore some satisfying, if stormy, entanglements with women. After her antidepressant response she got into her first "big romance" with a woman she had met at the Unitarian church. Life was pretty much trouble-free until about a year ago, when she fell into another funk just like the one her gynecologist treated. By this time Evelyn was seeing the nurse practitioner for her primary care needs, so she approached the NP and requested the same antidepressant as before.

Once again, the antidepressant was "a miracle," and this time, at her NP's suggestion, Evelyn resolved to stay with it. She was able to carry on with work, and she soon thereafter talked her partner into moving in with her, into a "fixer-upper" home she had coveted for years and bought on impulse. Evelyn had single-handedly gutted the spare bedroom, stripped the dining room wallpaper, sanded the floors, and had the kitchen halfway torn up when she "hit a wall" and lost interest in continuing any of it. Her relationship tanked, as she couldn't stand to be around anyone, even her partner. After the partner moved out, Evelyn went back to the NP, once again depressed. She did not think to mention the high-energy period that accompanied the purchase of the house. The NP told her the medication must have "pooped out" (stopped working) and prescribed a different one. The new one took a little longer to build up an effect, but eventually Evelyn was back to her old "hyper" self. She held on to it long enough to reconcile with her partner and to finish the kitchen renovation before the effect faded again. An increase in the dose brought back the energy and enthusiasm. She finished some old projects and started some new ones, but eventually she again fell into a funk, leaving a mess of half-finished home improvement projects. The NP wasn't willing to increase the antidepressant any further, as they were already at the maximum recommended dose.

Dr. Engel, on reviewing this story with Evelyn, wants to know more about these periods of high energy that followed the onset of antidepressant therapy and asks Evelyn about them. Specifically, were there any changes in her sleep, in the way she experienced her thoughts and spoke with other people, in her confidence? Evelyn could say yes to all of these. During those times when she was most energized, she could fool around with projects until one or two o'clock in the morning and still be fresh for work the next day. Her thoughts seemed to have a clarity she had never before known, and she felt strongly that she was right, all the time. Moreover, she had a lot of thoughts, tumbling over one another for her attention. It was exciting, especially when she could get someone to listen to all of her ideas. Dr. Engel asks if any of this caused trouble— did she take reckless risks, embarrass friends, commit herself to things she couldn't get out of? No, there didn't seem to be any downside to her upside, other than when the energy lapsed and she was left with a mess to clean up in whatever rooms she was renovating. (2)

Dr. Engel tells Evelyn that the problem with her treatment up to this point is that she has been treated for the wrong disorder. Evelyn has bipolar disorder, not major depressive disorder, and antidepressants do not effectively treat bipolar disorder. (3) Evelyn is highly skeptical. Dr. Engel explains that the times of high energy and enthusiasm were possibly manias and were certainly at least hypomanias. "But what's the problem with that? It's not like I'm spending myself bankrupt or sleeping around. I get a lot done. It beats the heck out of being depressed. Can't you find something that will help me stay up like that all the time?" Dr. Engel smiles wistfully but says, "I wish I had something like that; I could sell it myself and become a billionaire. The problem is not with the hypomanias themselves—they don't bother you or cause trouble and you find them stimulating—the problem is that having hypomanias means you won't respond to antidepressant therapy as well as you would if you only had depressive mood swings." (4)

"But I can't go on being depressed. I need an antidepressant, like today." Dr. Engel explains that an antidepressant might be indicated, but Evelyn's history has already established that an antidepressant on its own would not be a good choice, reminding her that the most recent episode occurred while she was already taking an antidepressant. (5) Dr. Engel agrees to give her an antidepressant so long as she also takes lithium, which has the strongest evidence for effectiveness at both treating and preventing manic and depressive mood swings in bipolar disorder.

As before, Evelyn mounts a rapid recovery after starting the antidepressant, but she also notices that she doesn't get quite as high as she did the last few times she started an antidepressant. She calls Dr. Engel to report she's "kinda bummed" about that, (6) and Dr. Engel counsels that, while she may miss the high points of her mood swings, she will not miss the low points, and her energy and motivation are likely to be more reliable if she stays with the lithium.

Months pass, and she is now seeing Dr. Engel every eight weeks. Although the good period lasts longer this time, her mood once again takes a dive, not long after her last appointment with Dr. Engel. It's not quite as bad as before and she's busy at work, but she considers making a call to try to get her next appointment moved up. Evelyn procrastinates, and within two weeks her mood has come back to baseline on its own, so she doesn't call. And then it dips again a month later and rises back to baseline over a few weeks, just before her next visit, when she reports only that she is feeling fine at the moment. Weeks later, as the third dip in three months begins to take hold, she makes an urgent visit to Dr. Engel to discuss going on a different antidepressant. (7) "This one isn't working any more. What's next?"

Dr. Engel makes a counterproposal that Evelyn initially finds rather unnerving: get rid of antidepressants altogether. She argues that she has had so much success getting out of depressions with antidepressants that she's afraid to not be on one, but Dr. Engel ventures that it seems likely the antidepressants may be making things worse, by counteracting the mood-stabilizing effects of lithium. Dr. Engel proposes that if she remains depressed after a few months, then they can try another antidepressant, provided she takes a second antimanic agent. She tapers from the antidepressant, still somewhat down, but it never gets to the point that she can't function. A month later she unexpectedly has another, milder but noticeable, dip in her mood and is able to ride it out. After six months on lithium alone, she does not notice any significant mood swings, but she still misses the "hyper." (8)

Summary: Bipolar Depression

··

- ▶ In between major depressive disorder and full-blown, unmistakable manic-depressive illness, there is a spectrum that encompasses a wide range of presentations of mood instability. Bipolar II—depressions with hypomanias—is probably the best known to psychiatrists currently, but one may also see other variants:
  - ▷ hyperthymic in youth (that is, irrepressible energy at baseline) but lapsing into depression in middle age
  - ▷ cyclothymic (moody without having full-severity manias or depressions)
  - ▷ manic mood swings only while taking antidepressants or stimulants
  - ▷ highly unstable moods that fluctuate from moment to moment
  - ▷ cycling into and out of depression without pushing above normal toward hypomania.
- ▶ Depression with bipolar disorder can be far trickier to treat than pure major depressive disorder. The clinician and the

patient both should bear in mind that mood stabilization is the top priority and that lasting relief from depression can only follow from having a stable mood.

▶ Long before a person recognizes moodiness as being an illness in need of treatment, those mood swings may become woven into the person's life story. The adventures and tragedies that in retrospect have obviously, to the observer, been driven by an abnormal mood state may seem in the moment to be just intense expressions of the human experience.

Case Notes

••

(1) The clue that there might be something more than major depressive disorder is Evelyn's family and social history. Her father's moodiness suggests the possibility of bipolar disorder, as does her own pattern of broken relationships, impulsive actions (like a brief Vegas marriage), and job instability.

(2) Mild manic (hypomanic) mood swings may also fail to arouse the concern of most people who have them; after all, they cause little, if any, trouble, and people are unlikely to seek medical help if feeling better than normal. To discover them, a physician often must ask directly about periods of elation, excitement, irritability, and restlessness combined with a diminished need for sleep and an increase in speech and activity. Anyone can have a few hours or a day like this, but more than a few days suggests bipolar disorder.

(3) "Poop outs"—depressions that recur after someone has responded to an antidepressant—arise for a variety of reasons both identifiable and obscure. Among the identifiable reasons are newly stressful situations, spotty adherence to treatment, and inadequate dosing. It may be more difficult, if not impos-

sible, to detect pseudoresponse (that is, treatment coinciding with a spontaneous remission from illness) and some forms of rapidly cycling bipolar spectrum disorder in which the patient never develops classic manic elation. In the latter case, an antidepressant may or may not have pushed the patient out of a depression, but it certainly failed to keep the patient from cycling into another one, or it possibly accelerated the mood cycling.

(4) Patients who have heard about bipolar disorder are often quick to deny that their own high periods are truly manic or signs of anything but a relief from depressive illness. Clinicians may have success in persuading patients that they have bipolar disorder (rather than depression) by reassuring the patient that the principal clinical significance of the hypomanic swings is not the hypomanias themselves, but rather that the hypomanias may signify the patient's likely unstable response to treatment for depression.

(5) Some people who have hypomanias with depression achieve the hoped-for antidepressant response, but many will find antidepressant effects to be either transient or inflammatory. For these individuals, the net result of being on an antidepressant is more depression, because there is more cycling into depression.

(6) Stabilization of the mood from bipolar disorder can also produce a demoralized state in which the patient finds that life without the driving force of hypomanias lacks luster and spark. It takes more effort to accomplish things that once came easily because of the bubbling energy level, and this stabilization leaves some people discouraged.

(7) The expected six- to eight-week delay in full antidepressant response means that it can never be proven whether a

person who cycles repeatedly into episodes of two months or less has responded to an antidepressant or has simply cycled spontaneously out of it. On this basis alone it makes little sense to give an antidepressant to a rapidly switching patient.

(8) It appears that Evelyn's cycling was made worse by the antidepressant, and she becomes less depressed (cycles less frequently into depression) when she is taken off antidepressants.

FRANCES

Overmedication

● ●

OVERVIEW: Frances has been treated with a variety of medications to try to manage her major depression, the specific
symptoms of depression that bother her the most, and the side
effects of the medications used to treat these problems. As a
result, she is clinically intoxicated and still feels down. Adding
more medications will make her more intoxicated, but fewer
might leave her suicidally depressed. After being admitted to a
psychiatric unit to be detoxed, Frances is sent home on a simpler
and more effective regimen of antidepressants, but no additional
medications for specific symptoms like anxiety or insomnia.

● ●

In the hall on the way back to the psychiatry office suite after
a bathroom break, Dr. Fender sidesteps an unsteady woman

59

who lumbers with a cane in one hand and the other touching the wall, and wonders idly how someone could be drunk so early in the day. Ten minutes later, the woman—Frances—is in the office, in search of "better meds for my bipolar disorder." Recalling how wobbly she appeared in the hallway, Dr. Fender first establishes that Frances does not intend to drive home; her son is waiting for her in the lobby.

Upon reviewing her history, Dr. Fender is surprised to learn that this dull-expressioned, slow-responding, fifty-something woman wearing sweats and with a tousled mound of hair, now slouching in the chair, has a PhD in astronomy and was running a local planetarium only a few years ago, until she was disabled by her mental illness. She hasn't touched alcohol in years. Otherwise, the story is hard to gather. Frances slurs, nods off a few times, gives vague and contradictory accounts of her life history and course of illness, and often misinterprets the point of a question. When asked to describe what her symptoms are like, she instead explains why they occur, often using psychiatric jargon, but with evident difficulty pinning down details. Concerned about her inability to provide a coherent history, Dr. Fender performs a screening test for cognitive functioning and finds that Frances scores in the "impaired" range. But, noting the sleepiness, slurred speech, and unsteady gait, Dr. Fender suspects delirium—an altered state of consciousness due to gross brain dysfunction—is the most pressing problem. (1)

Frances is here because her last psychiatrist encouraged her to find another psychiatrist. "Dr. Foulk gave up on me. My case was too tough. They said you were the best." She hands over a sheaf of papers: a copy of a set of progress notes from Dr. Foulk, along with pharmacy records. A quick skim through the computer-generated pharmacy record reveals at least twenty different psychiatric medications prescribed in various combinations over the past two years. The electronic progress notes from each monthly clinic visit with Dr. Foulk contain scant text and consist mostly of checklists for symptoms, mental status findings, diagnoses, and medications to be changed or renewed. (2) The verbal notes include:

- ▸ *More energy, but can't sleep due to racing thoughts. Plan: Check lithium level, increase bedtime antipsychotic, consider increase in antiepileptic mood stabilizer.*
- ▸ *Feels worse today. Can't concentrate. Plan: Increase antidepressant, add stimulant.*
- ▸ *Lowered antidepressant due to weight gain, but mood "crashed." Plan: Replace antidepressant.*

It is impossible from these cryptic notes to be certain that Frances has had a combination of enough symptoms of major depressive disorder at a minimum degree of severity for a long enough period of time to fully justify the diagnosis. Only a vague determination of whether she has improved or not (more often not) and which medication changes were being made is possible. (3) Dr. Fender sees in the record that Dr. Foulk was never able to discontinue a medication without adding another one.

"So tell me more about the bipolar disorder and anxiety that Dr. Foulk was unable to help you with."

Through painstaking interrogation, some educated guesswork, and, most importantly, calling the son into the office as an objective and clear-headed informant, Dr. Fender is able to piece together an idea about Frances's problems. She was doing fairly well until two years ago. Up to then she had occasional bouts of depression, never mania, but they generally went away on their own or, in a few cases, with the help of an antidepressant.

Two years ago, right after her divorce, she fell into a deep depression and was admitted to the hospital's psychiatry unit after an attempted suicide by overdose, which first put her in the intensive care unit for a few days. At the time of the psychiatry admission she was highly agitated, pacing until her feet were blistered, clawing at her skin, waking up at night screaming in anguish ("It was hell!" she recalls). The medical staff at the hospital interpreted the agitation as a symptom of bipolar disorder and put her on an antipsychotic, an anticonvulsant mood stabilizer, an antidepressant, and a benzodiazepine. After a week she was still down but calmer and no longer eager to kill herself. But in the subsequent months she never rebounded to the point where she felt able to go back to work. Her son came to stay with her as she spent increasing amounts of time on her couch, taking poor care of herself. She started seeing Dr. Foulk after the hospitalization, and despite all of Dr. Foulk's efforts she has continued to be disabled by depression.

Now, however, Frances no longer has the agitation that got her hospitalized. Instead, she struggles with persistent fatigue and inertia. She feels too tired to buy groceries, to do any housework, to go to church. She doesn't want to hear from friends, so she stopped checking her e-mail and voicemail messages. She gave her dog to a cousin because it was too much trouble to walk him. She wishes every day she would just not wake up, or that a meteor would fall through her roof, but insists she lacks the "guts" to take her own life. Although she doesn't prepare meals, she does gorge on snack foods, and she has managed to gain a bundle of fat around her middle ("*That* wasn't there two years ago, I assure you"). She complains that she can't sleep without her sleeping pills, but when asked to describe a typical night's sleep, reports that she's typically in bed by nine o'clock, struggles until about midnight to fall asleep, gets up at nine o'clock the next morning to eat something, goes back to sleep until around one o'clock in the afternoon, eats, watches TV, then naps for a few hours again in the late afternoon. (4)

"So that sounds like the depression part of the bipolar disorder. What about the manic?" asks Dr. Fender. Neither Frances nor her son can describe what she might have said to the psychiatrists during her hospital stay to warrant the diagnosis of bipolar disorder. When queried about specific symptoms of mania, she admits that she has at times experienced symptoms of irritability and "racing thoughts" that she describes as "going around and around about the same worries." She has never had a period of elated mood, excessive energy, diminished need to sleep, hypertalkativeness, or grandiosity. (5) She has also never had hallucinations, delusions, or other signs of psychosis.

Reviewing Frances's active medications, Dr. Fender establishes that she is currently taking two different second-generation neuroleptics (one at twice the normal dose used for someone with active hallucinations or delusions), lithium, an anticonvulsant, two antidepressants, two benzodiazepines along with another heavily advertised prescription sleeping pill, and two forms of stimulants. She is also taking a "muscle relaxant," an antivertigo drug, and a variety of medications for hypertension, diabetes, and cholesterol. (6) Dr. Fender responds, "I think you may be intoxicated from being on so many medications. I see in the notes that Dr. Foulk has tried to remove some of them from time to time, but ends up going back on them or replacing them with something else. What is going on at those times?"

Frances seems a bit perplexed by the question. "Well, I guess I just need them. If I don't take my sleeping pills, I'm awake half the night. If I don't take the anxiety pills, I get panic attacks. If I don't take the ADHD pills, I feel so foggy I can't even focus on a TV show...Dr. Foulk never let me leave the office without something to help me feel better."

Dr. Fender considers the options. Most, maybe all, the medications must be stopped in order to resolve the delirium, but there are significant risks. (7) Even with a good support system and strong therapeutic relationship with a physician, Frances might not be able to commit to a plan of medication simplification that could take months to unfold in an outpatient setting. It is doubtful that she would even remember in a week or two why she needs to lower her medications. The next best alternative might be a partial hospitalization or intensive outpatient program where the medications could be microman-aged and Frances's condition could be assessed every day. These programs are hard to find in the area, however, and would require Frances's son to take time off of work to ferry her to and from the program. "I think the best thing to do would be to admit you to the hospital, where you can have intensive support while we take you off as many of these medications as we can as quickly and safely as we can, and then start from scratch."

Frances is admitted to the psychiatry inpatient unit and, remarkably, is able to tolerate the rapid removal of all but a few of the psychiatric medications (keeping only the ones that must be tapered gradually). At worst, she suffers a couple of nights with erratic sleep and a couple of episodes of panic, which the nurses are able to talk her through. Within a week, she is off almost everything but her mood is no better, and she pleads to go back on some of the medications. Dr. Fender points out that a bit more time would be needed to establish which medications are likely to do more good than harm, and urges her to stay with the plan at least for another week. Dr. Fender acknowledges Frances's disappointment but adds that being no worse off and on fewer drugs is an unequivocal win, and promises to work closely with her until she is better.

After another week, with a small dose of benzodiazepine as the only psychiatric drug remaining, Frances has to admit that her thinking has cleared up and she doesn't feel the need to spend so much time in bed. She still notices that she has little stamina for exercise or reading, which she finds frustrating, but remarks that she has finally regained some hope that she can return to being active again in time. She would like to contact the planetarium to offer her services as a volunteer. Soon thereafter she is discharged home.

Six months later and recovered to the point that she gets out of the house daily to volunteer or run errands or visit friends, Frances notices a growing drag on her spirits and energy, progressing to sleeplessness and a sense that she has to push herself to do things that were easy a few weeks before. She sees Dr. Fender and requests sleeping pills, a stimulant, and something for anxiety, but she is willing to accept Dr. Fender's counteroffer of an antidepressant and weekly visits until she is feeling better. While it takes a fair amount of coaxing and counseling to stick with this conservative medication plan, Frances returns to feeling normal in a matter of weeks, without sacrificing her growing constellation of activities. (8)

Summary: Overmedication
....

▸ Depression cannot be diagnosed accurately or treated effectively if the person has delirium.

▶ The power, efficiency, and ever-broadening variety of modern psychotropic medications have increased the risk that the treatments themselves, if applied overzealously, can cause delirium and thus create more problems than they solve.

▶ It generally takes far more time and effort to remove a medication of uncertain benefit than to add or switch a medication. Therefore physicians should be careful to establish that every current medication has a measurable benefit before adding any new ones.

▶ Success in the collaboration between a suffering patient and a well-meaning physician can be elusive if the physician reacts to problems by adding or switching medications without taking time to talk and support the patient through a bad patch.

Case Notes

••

(1) Delirium is a disturbance of consciousness that can affect cognitive and emotional functioning; it is brought about by some gross disruption of brain activity. Intoxication due to alcohol or illicit drug use is a common and familiar form of delirium, as is the loss of coherence that can occur in someone with a fever or other serious systemic medical illness. It is quite possible to worsen the condition of a person with delirium by prescribing medications that affect brain functioning, such as antidepressants, antianxiety drugs, and even antipsychotic drugs. Antihistamines can be particularly harmful in this regard.

(2) The modern electronic medical record systematically records clinical information and has the useful virtues of permanence and portability; the chart cannot be lost (provided

the computer system is operating normally), and records can be printed or shared between physicians with the push of a button. But because the software interface used to capture and present the clinical data is generally based on clicking and unclicking buttons, these records suffer from the limitation of often including little useful textual information about the thought processes behind clinical decisions.

(3) One unfortunate side effect of the success of modern psychiatric medications is that the typical psychiatric visit has been reduced to a fifteen- to twenty-minute (or less) medication check, or "med check," on a monthly (or even less frequent) basis even when the patient is not doing well. This might be enough time to manage a more or less stable problem, but it is not nearly enough time to troubleshoot a problem in someone who is not responding well to treatment. Many a therapeutic impasse might be resolved without the need for a second opinion consultation were the physician or patient to insist on longer or more frequent visits to talk about the reasons why treatment is not working, and to work out individualized solutions.

(4) When the clinician examines the structure of the typical day of a person dragged down by depression or other mental disorder, a wealth of highly useful information emerges that cannot be gained merely from asking about symptoms and side effects. An hour-by-hour summary of daily activities not only helps the patient and physician take a hard look at how the patient is structuring his or her time, but also provides a template for future efforts to reintroduce structure into a life disorganized by mental illness.

(5) There is little evidence here to support the diagnosis of bipolar disorder. The only manic or hypomanic symptoms

are irritability and agitation (in the intensive care unit), which can also be a symptom of depression or delirium, and "racing thoughts," a phrase commonly used to indicate both the classic rapid manic cacophony of ideas and, as in this case, anxious ruminations or worries. The erroneous diagnosis of bipolar disorder underscores the importance for both clinician and patient of communicating in plain language rather than using medical jargon that may mean something different to the patient than it does to the clinician.

(6) Polypharmacy—the prescribing of multiple medications to address a problem—can be beneficial for difficult psychiatric problems, provided the benefits of each medication can be documented. But despite complaints about insomnia, a person who sleeps twelve to fourteen hours a day needs fewer, not more, sedating drugs. When addressing neurological or psychiatric complaints in someone taking multiple psychopharmaceuticals, the clinician should always consider the possibility that the underlying cause of the problem may be medication side effects that mimic the condition the medications are intended to be treating.

(7) Removing medications to treat the problem of medication-induced delirium can entail risk. First, the removal itself can create withdrawal symptoms; for antidepressants, these symptoms can be highly unpleasant, though they are seldom, if ever, dangerous. Second, and more unpredictably, the removal of a medication thought to be ineffective may reveal that in fact it was working to some extent, and its removal thus brings about a recurrence of symptoms. If side effects of withdrawal or a recurrence of symptoms become an obstacle to reducing the medication load for a delirious person, then the clinician may well consider and suggest admitting the person

to a partial hospital or inpatient psychiatric unit to adjust and regulate medications.

(8) It appears that at the time the medications were withdrawn Frances was not in an active state of major depressive disorder, but a new episode, warranting antidepressant treatment, emerged half a year later.

III : DEPRESSION-PLUS

In each of these three stories there is no question that the patient has had a major depressive episode. The problem is that symptoms of depression persist despite appropriate antidepressant therapy.

GARY

Double Depression

OVERVIEW: Gary has a history of severe depressions superimposed on a chronic low mood dating back to childhood, and he is stuck in life. Antidepressant medications have helped him out of the worst episodes but haven't touched his chronic sense of dissatisfaction. A comprehensive look at his life history suggests that his chronic low mood pre-dates his major depressive episodes and perseveres even when he is functioning relatively well. The chronically low mood can in turn be attributed to his upbringing in a grim household that reinforced an innate temperamental tendency to prioritize avoiding pain over pursuing pleasure. Psychotherapy in addition to medication helps him move ahead with life, but it's not clear that he feels much better.

"I'm never *not* depressed," says Gary, the neatly groomed, forty-ish man in Dr. Gavin's office. "I think about suicide every day. On a good day I can put it out of my mind and get on with my business. On a bad day, the idea that I could put an end to my misery gives me comfort...but I don't think I'd ever go through with it."

Gary appears oddly animated for someone who thinks about suicide every day. Dr. Gavin guesses out loud, "So would this be one of your good days?"

Gary loses his subtle smile. "Well, that's really the problem now. It's getting harder to tell whether I'm having a good day or a bad day." Dr. Gavin takes this ambiguous statement as a cue to probe Gary's history. Gary was a longtime patient of Dr. Gavin's psychopharmacologist colleague, Dr. Glenn, who is nearing retirement. The two doctors have discussed Gary's case by phone, so Dr. Gavin has some vague idea about Gary's story, but Dr. Glenn's chicken-scratch handwriting makes the copy of the clinic records that accompanied the referral almost useless.

Gary is an accountant in a midlevel job at a state agency. He has never married. He's in a relationship with a woman but spends far more time with his aging parents, who live nearby in the same house where Gary grew up. His father is a retired firefighter, and his mother stayed at home with Gary and his older sister. Sadly, his sister died in her teens from cancer. The parents have struggled with medical problems, mostly cardiovascular and pulmonary issues. "They haven't taken very good care of themselves," Gary says. They seem to need Gary's help on an almost daily basis with shopping, driving to doctor appointments, fixing things around the house, and so on. Gary notes that his parents both seem depressed. They don't appear to have any outside interests and spend much of their time "watching the news and arguing. They've always been like that." Neither has been treated for depression. Gary has suggested it but was met with firm refusals.

Gary saw a psychologist while in his teens, briefly, after his sister died. He believes now that he was depressed long before that. He was an isolated, quietly unhappy child. He could never see the point of running around with the other neighborhood kids, and he was never much good at sports, so he stopped trying after middle school. Academics came easily. He was the kid who always knew the answer to the teacher's question but wouldn't raise his hand. In groups he was innocuous enough to be tolerated, only rarely the butt of jokes or bullying, content to hover on the margins. He spent his free time on solitary hobbies. Gary amassed collections of stamps, comic books, and rocks. He built plastic models and read epics of fantasy literature. "I can't say I ever really had fun, but it felt good if I could find a rare stamp." His social life improved dramatically in high school, as he began to discover other kids with interests akin to his, but for the most part they also shared a common aversion to "fun" and spent long hours of free time hanging out, participating in fantasy role-play games, or listening to music. He did not date in high school—he had never had enough of an itch for romance to overcome his fear of certain rejection.

He and his high school pals had discussed suicide often, mostly as a fantasy or philosophical topic. One girl in his social group started cutting herself with a razor and took a serious overdose junior year, and after that she changed schools. They never heard from her again. He had always found the suicide discussions fascinating in the abstract but had never felt a desire to end his life "until I went off to college."

The first month of college, Gary explains, was "actually the

best time in my life. The first time I knew what 'fun' meant."
He shared interests with a sizable group of peers and felt like
he could relate to almost everyone he met. He started to attend
campus concerts and mixers with girls, and to feel he might
soon work himself up to asking one out on a date. "And then
October hit...no, it ran me over." One morning, he recalls, he
had simply lost the will to get out of bed and go to class. The
early freshman froth had evaporated, leaving him with the
feeling that it was all pointless, everybody was phony, and the
best possible endpoint of academic success would make him a
"slave to the machine."

He assumed at first that the gloom would pass and that
he would get back his academic drive, but the longer he stayed
away from class, the more comfortable he felt holed up in his
room. Gary became increasingly uneasy about venturing out.
He tried to manage by studying without going to class, but "it
was like my textbooks had all been rewritten in Russian"—he
could spend hours trying to read one page and understand
nothing from it—so he gave up trying. The communal shower
meant close encounters with other floor residents, so he
avoided bathing. For six weeks he stayed in his dorm room
virtually all the time. By the third week his roommate had peti-
tioned for and was granted a new residential placement, leaving
Gary contentedly alone.

Gary developed a routine of leaving his room once a day
for a meal—his appetite was nearly nonexistent—and once a
week he went to the campus library to check out an armful of
graphic novels. That was about all the energy he could muster.
The graphic novels distracted him from his intrusive fantasies
of jumping from the roof of the dorm or hanging himself in his
room or stealing his father's gun and shooting himself in the

woods. Ashamed of his dirty, inactive state and the deceptions he was using to maintain it, he assured anyone who came to check on him that he was fine and needed no help, and said the same to his parents on the rare occasion he accepted a phone call. (1)

The reckoning came at the end of the semester, when he had to admit to his parents that he had no grades, as he had effectively dropped all his classes. They took him to his old pediatrician back home, who wasn't quite sure what to make of Gary's problem and so referred him to a child psychiatrist who diagnosed depression and recommended psychotherapy. Over a few months the suicidal thoughts ebbed, and he gradually found his way back to being the solitary, somewhat nihilistic person he had been in high school. He had no desire to return to college (and his parents were wary of paying the tuition), so he stayed home and took classes at the local community college.

He limped along in this fashion for several more years, socially inert but keeping to a disciplined routine the therapist had instilled in him, slowly accumulating credits before hitting another, "darker" wave of depression similar to what had upended his freshman year away at college. He called his old therapist, but this time the therapist recommended he seek psychiatric help in addition to restarting therapy. With some trepidation Gary agreed, was placed on an antidepressant, and began to feel better than he had felt since that first month of college. He dropped out of therapy, as it no longer seemed necessary, and stayed on the antidepressant. Over the subsequent year he transferred his credits to a four-year university nearby, found a job, moved out of his parents' home and into his own apartment, rekindled some old friendships, and started dating his present girlfriend. Eventually he graduated—a bit later than expected, but with good enough credentials to land an account-ing post in the state government, his present job.

And there things have remained, more or less, for over a decade. (2) He and the girlfriend (also treated for depression) are no closer to marrying or starting a family—or for that matter to breaking up and finding more satisfying partners—than they were ten years ago. Despite encouragement from his supervisors, Gary lacks the ambition to seek a promotion; meanwhile he has grown bored with number crunching and resentful of younger colleagues leapfrogging him into higher-status positions. His interests revolve around a few solitary hobbies that fuel his only regular social contact, Internet-based discussion groups. He has no real joy and can imagine nothing to be fun, yet he can occasionally become energized by an impending comics convention or by some acquisition for one of his collections. (3)

He started seeing Dr. Glenn soon after getting the state job and the health insurance coverage that came with it. Dr. Glenn and Gary have tried a variety of methods to try to recover that fleeting feeling of generalized happiness Gary had the first month away at college, but with no success. Raising the antidepressant dose above the standard guidelines only gave him more side effects. Trying to wean from antidepressants altogether triggered a slip into the deeper sort of depression. Combinations and switches of medications have made Gary's life no better and sometimes have made it worse.

"Dr. Glenn was pretty old-school," says Gary. "I have this fantasy that you might have something new to get me out of this rut, but I expect it will be just more of the same."

Dr. Gavin replies, "I don't think there's a simple, quick-and-easy fix, but I think there may be a way to make life better for you. It starts with sorting out the different ways depression affects you." Dr. Gavin observes that Gary seems to have two different kinds of depression. The deeper depressions that have upended his life at times and that emerge when he goes too low on his antidepressant have all the hallmarks of a recurrent major depressive disorder. Treating these depressions with the right medication has reliably permitted a full return to work, interests, and relationships such as they are—a basically successful, if constricted, degree of adult adjustment. (4)

But the other depression that constricts his quality of life—the persistent low mood that has been there since childhood—has proven harder to resolve. Dr. Gavin conjectures that chronic low mood—dysthymia—in someone who has had episodes of full-blown depression sometimes indicates that the major depressive disorder has been undertreated. While that might still be the case for Gary, thus far there has been no additional success from trying to boost antidepressant medications, so it may be time to test the second hypothesis: that Gary's chronic depression is something other than a partially treated major depressive disorder.

"But what else could it be?" Gary asks, with some impatience. "Are you suggesting that I'm just unhappy with life? That I need to try harder? You just said I had a 'successful adjustment,' whatever that means. So then what in the world could I change that would make me any happier?" (5)

"Let's back up a bit. No, I don't think you just need to 'try harder' or that there's any particularly demoralizing aspect to your life that could be fixed that would make things right. But from everything you've told me, it sounds like you are profoundly unhappy with life—not discontented in some trivial or superficial way, but constitutionally unhappy. I've just met you today, so I don't think I know enough about you to explain everything, but as a working hypothesis, I believe your chronic, constitutional unhappiness is a consequence of several different forces.

"First, you told me that you thought your parents were depressed. That suggests to me the possibility that life at home when you were growing up might have been kind of drab and lifeless."

"Yeah...okay. We weren't like one of those sitcom families on TV, but who is?"

"You didn't have much of a basis to compare, since you didn't have a lot of friends, and didn't see other kids' families in action."

Gary pondered, "I remember we used to have fun when we'd visit my aunt and uncle on holidays. My uncle used to play tricks, like 'finding' a nickel in my ear. Always a lot of games and funny stories and camping indoors in the basement with sleeping bags and watching TV half the night. Even the food was fun—they had the kinds of sugary cereals my parents wouldn't buy. I always assumed they were just trying hard to be sociable. So maybe they were like that all the time, not just when they had company?"

"Perhaps. And as for the atmosphere at your house, I imagine losing your sister didn't help." Gary nodded. "Now, of course, none of that means you were destined to be an unhappy adult, but it made it harder because, as you said yourself, you really didn't understand the meaning of 'fun' until that brief period after you started college."

"And then right after that the bottom fell out."

"Right. And without even thinking about it directly, that

experience might have taught you an unfortunate lesson—that suffering is the inevitable consequence of happiness. Why make an effort or take chances to achieve more happiness when depression can come along and steal it away? None of this means you were doomed to be unhappy. There are plenty of people with major depressive disorder who enjoy life perfectly well when they're not depressed."

"You said that before…okay, maybe I never learned how to be happy because I was raised in a home with unhappy people, and maybe life taught me that any happiness you do find is fleeting and not worth it because depression can take it away. But you're also saying some people could be happy despite those things. Why not me? Why am I always doomed to be depressed?" (6)

"Good question. Maybe the best way to explain it is to think about how people can vary. Some people are tall, some people are short, some people are smart, others not so much. Some people are outgoing and have fun easily, others are reserved and get more satisfaction from the quieter pleasures of life."

"The second one, that sounds like me."

"And even that doesn't mean that you're doomed to unhappiness, just that in your case, if you are indeed a person who doesn't find it easy to feel happy, and who was raised in circumstances that did not prepare you to be creative in finding ways to improve your happiness, and then struck with an illness that shook your faith that happiness is even real or possible—well…"

"So meds aren't going to help with that."

"Not much, except in keeping the major depression away and allowing you to start looking for ways to improve your happiness with some confidence that you'll be able to keep it up when you do find them. For the rest of it, I think there's a lot to be gained from psychotherapy." (7)

With Dr. Gavin's help and ongoing management of major depressive disorder, Gary finds a therapist with whom he feels comfortable, and over several years they work on these issues. At the end of psychotherapy treatment, Gary is not certain whether it helped, but he no longer thinks of suicide, has made good progress toward his master's degree and has kindled a promising new relationship with someone he met in his MBA program. (8)

Summary: Double Depression

- ▸ "Double depression" is a psychiatric colloquialism that used to denote major depressive disorder superimposed on dysthymic disorder or depressive personality. The term in use currently is "persistent depressive disorder."
- ▸ There are constitutionally gloomy people who never lapse into a major depressive episode, and there are cheerful people who occasionally fall into major depression. These are separate problems that can interact when both are present. When a gloomy person has had major depressive disorder, the gloomy personality can easily be mistaken for a manifestation of the major depressive disorder.
- ▸ A constitutionally gloomy person recovering from major depression is likely to recover back to a state of gloominess; one cannot take the low mood alone as the key indicator of undertreated major depressive disorder.
- ▸ Major depressive disorder is defined as a disorder by its adverse impact on functioning. Not every person with major depressive disorder becomes incapacitated; many

will heroically drag themselves out of bed and force themselves to go to work. But if you look at their productivity, or
how efficiently they can do what they were able to do before
they had depression, you will see a tangible decline in
function. The ability of a person with chronically low mood
to sustain a job and relationships over many years, however
unsatisfying they are, does not prove, but does suggest,
that the low mood stems from something other than major
depressive disorder.

Case Notes

(1) Here is another variation of the major depressive
syndrome. Gary's symptoms are similar to but not identical
to those of other people with major depressive disorder, while
his response to the illness—going with it rather than fighting
it—appears to emerge from enduring qualities in his individual
character.

(2) One of the essential features of major depressive
disorder, beyond the symptoms, is the fact that it significantly
impairs functioning. The episode in college clearly impaired
Gary's functioning. When the psychiatrist analyzed his apparent failed treatment response, the critical observation that
differentiated major depressive disorder from some other cause
of low mood was that, after starting antidepressants, Gary was
able to function steadily despite persistently complaining of low
mood.

(3) "Persistent depressive disorder" is a diagnosis now in
use in psychiatry to replace the term "dysthymia." Both terms
refer to a chronic, "low-grade"—that is, relatively mild—depressive state. By definition, these states do not cause the same
degree of impairment as major depressive disorder, and they go

on for years at a time with little respite. The major difference between them is that someone with persistent depressive disorder might have episodes of major depressive disorder along with the persistent, milder state of depression, while in the old system someone who had dysthymia along with episodes of major depressive disorder would have been diagnosed as having major depressive disorder, not dysthymia.

(4) The critical question is whether the depressive symptoms between the "darker" episodes are an attenuated form of the depressive state that is due to a malfunctioning brain, or whether they constitute a different problem: a depressive trait that comes from a brain that functions perfectly well but is poorly attuned to the environment in which it finds itself.

(5) Psychiatrists once diagnosed "neurotic depression" and "depressive personality disorder," but these constructs fell by the wayside many years ago in favor of "dysthymic disorder." Is there such a thing as a "depressive personality"? Are some people simply predisposed by nature to gloominess? While on the one hand most of us can think of individuals who might fit that description, on the other hand the implication that depression is woven into a personality as a permanent feature could also be taken as overly pessimistic about the prospect of improvement for the person.

(6) What to make of patients whose only persistent symptom of depression is low mood? As a matter of temperament, some people are easily distressed and others are imperturbable; those in the former group might not feel down all the time, but under any given circumstance, positive or negative, they will suffer more psychological pain than the average person. A success for the person with a depressive temperament therefore may bring not joy but angst that it was undeserved

or that later failure is inevitable. Such a person would be most content within a bubble that prevents change in either positive or negative directions, if not for the prospect of suffering from frustration associated with stagnation.

(7) The clinician's first step in helping patients with a depressive disposition is to reduce expectations that the standard treatments that are so effective for major depressive disorder are likely to be as successful in alleviating the chronic low mood. Reducing expectations frees the person from the burden of believing that the chronic depressions are a sign of treatment (or personal) failure. Psychotherapy won't change the depressive temperament, but it may at least allow the patient to assess the ups and downs of life objectively and not by reference to emotions that consistently bias negative.

(8) The implication here is that Gary has certainly benefited from psychotherapy in terms of love and work, but that the pace of psychotherapy can influence the patient's psychological growth so slowly that it appears as though psychological growth happened of its own accord.

HANNAH

Depressed Functioning

OVERVIEW: Hannah is a young adult living with her parents. She has suffered from major depression. Not only has she made no progress in life since high school, but she has also regressed to a state of near inertia. Outwardly she looks almost the same whether she is in a severe depression or in the chronic, moderate depression she complains of most of the time. But a close look at her symptoms suggests the chronic, moderate depression may be more of a pervasive demoralization reinforced by her state of learned helplessness. A rehabilitative approach to directly address her functional debilitation, combined with medication management for depression, gets her moving toward independence.

Hannah, age 25, sits quietly in Dr. Hernandez's office while her mother does most of the talking. Dr. Hernandez, who has a local reputation as an expert in mood disorders, has been asked to see Hannah for a second opinion consultation.

"Hannah's been depressed ever since middle school. Can you help us?" The word "us" immediately triggers the doctor's concerns about parent-child enmeshment, but Dr. Hernandez sets that concern aside for the moment to explore how Hannah got to this point.

Hannah is the youngest of four children of a factory foreman and a saleswoman in a department store, who tells Dr. Hernandez: "I had the baby blues after my first three, but after Hannah I was truly crazy—I had awful, awful thoughts about killing myself and the kids so I checked myself into the hospital." (1) Hannah's mother recovered but struggled with depressions throughout Hannah's early years until the psychiatrist found the right combination of medications. During the rough times, Hannah's grandmother would look after the children.

Hannah's father "goes off to his man cave, drinks beer, and watches sports all weekend. He's not very involved with us." Hannah's three siblings are out of the house and fairly stable; two have been treated for depression and anxiety problems. Hannah's mother mentions that some of her own siblings have been depressed, but they don't have a close relationship and so she doesn't know the details. A cousin on Hannah's mother's side committed suicide a few years ago, and Hannah's maternal grandmother had dementia and was depressed at the end of her life. She spent her last years living in Hannah's household and died when Hannah was a teenager.

Hannah was not an unhappy child, but "boy, could she throw a tantrum!" She had loud, uncontrollable screaming fits about once a month. "There was no way she was going to day care. She'd cry when I dropped her off, and she'd cry all day. Finally I had to quit work and stay home with her." The transition to school was not much better. "I had to stay in the classroom with her for the first few weeks until she got used to it." (2)

School was never Hannah's strong suit; she had minimal interest, did nominal work, made mediocre grades. She signed up to play the French horn in the school orchestra and was in Brownies and Girl Scouts. She tended to have one close girlfriend at a time, with whom she would "hang out" until they had the inevitable fight. Hannah went through friendships like this about every other year.

Hannah first showed a "dark side" in seventh grade, around the time her ailing grandmother came to stay with the family. A friend introduced her to Goth culture, and Hannah continued to wear dark clothing and bleak makeup long after that friendship broke up. She began to press her mother to let her get her ears pierced and her mother finally signed on, ultimately agreeing to multiple ear piercings, "but I wouldn't go for her getting pierced anywhere else."

"And then one day I hear this scream and see all this bloody tissue, and she's crying and holding ice on her nose—she had tried to pierce her own nose."

"Well, you wouldn't let me get it done," Hannah interjects. The piercing caused an infection and left a small scar. Dr. Hernandez looks hard at Hannah's nose and can barely see a tiny bump on the left side of her nostril. "Then she started to disappear from the table after dinner, and I'd hear noises like she was throwing up, but she said she was fine."

"I stopped her from going to the bathroom right after meals, but then she started cutting herself." Hannah's mother had been slow to catch on to this behavior at first, until she began to notice bandages on Hannah's arms and thighs that covered up rows of fine cuts in her skin. (3)

Dr. Hernandez asks Hannah, "Why did you cut yourself?" She responds, "I wanted to punish myself and, besides, it made me feel less tense. Also, I was getting tired of throwing up. When I would cut myself, I wouldn't feel like throwing up anymore." Hannah's mother recounts Hannah's tearful complaints at the time, that she hated life, that she was ugly and stupid, and that the "hideous" scar on her nose and plummeting grades only proved she was right.

Hannah then saw a child psychologist who tried to get her to remember who had sexually abused her in the past. Hannah could never recall anything like that, and her mother thought it was impossible because Hannah was never alone with anyone except girlfriends. But the therapist kept insisting that Hannah should undergo hypnosis to help her remember. Eventually Hannah became annoyed with the therapist, and stopped going.

A different psychologist suggested that Hannah might have depression and referred them to a child psychiatrist. The psychiatrist, Dr. Hobart, confirmed the diagnosis and prescribed an antidepressant. "I wasn't so sure about that at first," Hannah's mother explains, "I didn't want her to take drugs, but the doctor showed me a video about teenage depression, and one of the kids reminded me of Hannah. Anyway, Hannah was okay with going on medication, so we started the antidepressant." Hannah's mother was pleasantly surprised to see Hannah gradually come back to her old self. She was able to catch up in school, she worked with a therapist to control her bulimic behavior, and there were no further cuts or bloody tissues in the bathroom.

"When my mom—her gramma—passed," Hannah's

mother added, "I was sure Hannah would fall apart, but she didn't. She just cried like the rest of us and got on with school."

Hannah's mother balked when Hannah wanted to stop the antidepressant the summer before high school ("she thought it was making her fat, but she wasn't fat."). Dr. Hobart approved the plan, however, and for a while she was none the worse without the antidepressant. Freshman and sophomore years went fairly smoothly.

About midway through junior year, Hannah says, "the black cloud returned." She stopped caring about school, friends, or any other activities; she wanted to sleep all the time; her grades slipped. Hannah's mother remembers vividly how surly Hannah was with anyone and everyone. The household supply of alcohol seemed to be disappearing, with Hannah as the likely culprit, and the smell of her clothes made it evident that she had taken up smoking cigarettes. Hannah admitted to both vices but resisted going back into treatment. "I didn't see the point of it. It wasn't me—I thought it was the world that was all messed up. But my mom wouldn't shut up about it, so I went back to Hobart and started back on meds."

Again the medications worked, and Hannah was able to keep up her grades and a few social activities through the end of the year. She scored surprisingly well on the college entrance exam and was encouraged by a school guidance counselor to apply to some four-year colleges. She wound up receiving a good financial aid package at a college in a neighboring state. But despite being stable on the antidepressant, by the second half of senior year she had serious doubts about going off to college. She requested and received a one-year deferment.

"I thought she would want to earn some money, maybe have a little fun, travel, I don't know, before she went off to college, and we were willing to support her, but she didn't want to do anything!" After graduation, Hannah quickly fell into a pattern of getting up around midday, grabbing some cereal or toast or leftovers from the fridge and retreating to her room, closing the door, and "then she'd hide away until I begged her to come out to help with some housework or to have dinner with us. After dinner, she's back in her room. I could hear her moving around at all hours of the night." Hannah disagrees, adding that she usually takes her sleeping pills at midnight and is asleep by two o'clock, "not all hours of the night," Hannah argues back.

Life for Hannah and her parents has changed little over the past seven years. Despite being in constant psychiatric treatment and on medication, she felt no more ready to start college after a yearlong deferment than she did initially, so she withdrew from the four-year college. Her forays into adult life have been few and far between. She has enrolled in some community college classes but dropped as many as she completed. She has been on dates with boys she knew from high school or met on the Internet, but never with one more than a few times, and none at all in three years. "Finally, after we had to threaten to cut off her Internet, she got the part-time job at the animal shelter, and she's kept it for almost a year."

"Over a year, Mom, as of last week."

At this point, Dr. Hernandez shows Hannah's mother to the waiting room in order to talk with Hannah one on one. Hannah has filled out a symptom checklist, and Dr. Hernandez reviews the symptoms of major depression as she has reported them. Hannah's mood is "unhappy." She checks off that she has low motivation and doesn't enjoy anything. Asked further about that, Hannah explains that her friends are all married or working or moved away, so "there's no one to have any fun with." Asked what she does alone in her room so much of the time, she replies, "Oh, I dunno. Read a little. Binge-watch shows online. Play some poker."

"Poker?"

"Internet poker. I'm addicted. Small stakes, but it gives me a rush when I win."

Going through more symptoms, Hannah has checked off boxes for feeling tired, having an increase in weight ("probably because I don't exercise"), not sleeping (probed further, she explains that without her sleeping pills she would be up until at least four in the morning), being maybe a little guilty. (4) "Guilty?" Dr. Hernandez asks. "Yeah. Don't tell my mom this, but I do feel a little guilty about being such a sponge." Hannah has not experienced psychomotor agitation or retardation. She has left the question about suicidal ideation blank. She explains, "I'm not suicidal anymore, but I want to keep my options open."

Dr. Hernandez presses her to describe her past suicidal feelings. She identifies a few incidents. The first one, about two years after she graduated from high school, led her to take an overdose of an over-the-counter sleep aid. "Actually, I'm not sure I was really suicidal, but they kept telling me it must have been a suicide attempt, so I dunno. I was just feeling really frustrated and it wasn't going away, for weeks, so I finally thought what the hell, at least I'll relax. I guess it was called a suicide attempt because I really didn't care if I woke up or not. But it was only a dozen pills or so. I can't say I was serious about wanting to die."

At the time, Hannah recalls further, her mood wasn't just unhappy as it is now, it was "rock bottom." She stayed in bed all the time and stopped taking showers or getting dressed. She didn't care about eating and actually lost weight, "which wasn't so bad, I guess." She recalls that some of her friends were still around in those days, but she didn't answer their calls or texts. She stopped visiting her social media sites or updating her status. She adds, "I was really kind of worthless." (5)

Her parents found her in a semicomatose state after the overdose and had her hospitalized. She remained only a few days and was released on a combination of an antidepressant and an antipsychotic to try to make her feel "less frustrated." "Amazingly," she adds, "I actually had a brief period where I felt like I could get out of my rut and get a job and a place of my own and start dating, but it only lasted a few weeks." She adds, when asked, that this was the only time she had that good of a response to medication. (6)

With further probing, Dr. Hernandez establishes that there have been two other extended periods in the past seven years when her mood was about as low, when she wished she could just die quietly without hurting her parents, and she stopped having interest in television shows or poker or social media. Her therapist had convinced her to speak up when she feels like this, because each time it has led to a tweak of her medications and an improvement back to her usual state: low functioning but intact capacity for self-amusement. (7)

At the conclusion of the consultation, Dr. Hernandez calls Hannah's mother back into the room, explaining, "It's easier to remember all the important parts of the advice if more than one person hears it."

Dr. Hernandez begins by agreeing with the primary psychiatrist's diagnosis that Hannah has recurrent major depressive disorder, experienced as those times when she feels "rock bottom," stops doing anything for pleasure, and no longer cares whether she lives or dies. Nor is there any disagreement that she suffers from some form of low mood in between the more severe episodes of major depression. Dr. Hernandez explains that the diagnosis for this problem used to be called dysthymic disorder, but in the new diagnostic system it is now called persistent depressive disorder.

"You don't seem to have a big problem recovering from the worse periods of depression; on the few occasions they have happened, changing a medication or two has gotten back to your baseline. So the big question remains," Dr. Hernandez goes on, "what is this chronic depression that doesn't get better, and what can we do about it?" Hannah and her mother nod attentively.

"The goal of antidepressant treatment is not to bring a person to a state of total contentment. It is to allow the person to feel satisfied with the everyday activities of life: work, play, and relationships. What I hear from you," Dr. Hernandez goes on, "is that when you recover from severe depression, you recover into a situation that would make anyone unhappy: living with your parents and having no social life, no intimate relationships, no job, no sense of purpose or role to play or opportunity to do anything that might make life satisfying. Even if I had a wonder drug that could take away all the biological traces of depression but you continued living the way you do now, you would still consider yourself depressed." Hannah begins to fidget impatiently, "Even now, at your best, you continue to feel depressed most of the time because you're not really doing anything you can feel happy about. You'd like to be able to do those things, but they are not available to you. But when you're in the worse periods of depression, you wouldn't want to do them even if you could."

"How did she get this way, doctor?" her mother asks. "When she was a kid, she used to get all the way better from depression."

"True," Dr. Hernandez responds, "and I think the best explanation I can offer is that Hannah's ability to recover easily from depression was greatly helped by being able to return to a highly structured environment and expectations, namely, school. After she graduated from high school, there were no longer any set demands or structure, and she lacked either the opportunity or know-how or drive or discipline to impose on herself a new structure. Structure—that is, daily scheduled activities, roles with some responsibility attached to them, rewards for performing, and consequences for not perform-ing—is still what she needs, more than ever." (8)

"Umm," Hannah says, "but I can't—"

Dr. Hernandez interjects, "Let me stop you right there. I don't believe you 'can't.' I believe progress is extremely *difficult* for you, but not that you *can't* progress. I'll grant that, from your perspective, it may have taken as much or more brute willpower for you to take on that part-time job as it was for me to go to medical school for four years. But that doesn't mean you *can't* do more. It means that you need a different kind of help in order to be able to do more." (9)

Hannah glares doubtfully while her mother responds, "Don't you think Hannah will do more when she starts feeling better?"

"No, quite the contrary, I think Hannah will *feel* better

when she starts *doing* more. But, again, I don't want to minimize the challenge, or make it sound like I think it's just a matter of Hannah simply trying harder or willing it to happen. I think it's going to be a very big challenge, that she will need to learn new ways to motivate herself and to cope with stress, and that to make steady progress she will have to find a ready supply of courage."

"So what are you suggesting we do?" Hannah's mother asks.

Dr. Hernandez lays out an outline for a course of treatment, focusing on a rehabilitative model with cognitive behavioral therapy and life coaching. "For Hannah to function a lot better and derive more satisfaction from life, first she has to function just a little better, and once that becomes easier, to build on that." Turning to Hannah, "You've already taken an important step by getting that job at the animal shelter. It probably seemed extremely hard at first, but it's a lot easier now that you've done it for a year. Do you think you could maybe work two hours more every week?"

"Well, I have worked extra, when they needed me, but then I went back to my usual eight hours a week."

"So, you see, it is doable. But you're going to need a lot of encouragement to be sure you continue to make progress and overcome any barriers. A good behavioral therapist or a life coach will help. And of course you and your psychiatrist have to keep the bad depressions under control."

Hannah looks skeptical as they leave the consultation and shakes hands warily with Dr. Hernandez. Aside from a short thank-you e-mail from the referring psychiatrist, Dr. Hernandez hears no more about the case until receiving an e-mail from Hannah a year and a half later.

Dear Dr. Hernandez,

You probably don't remember me, but I saw you last year with my mom. I'm doing much better! But like you said, it hasn't been easy! I started with CBT like you suggested and it was slow going at first, but I started coming up with all these negative thoughts that were keeping me from trying new things, and it seemed to get easier and easier to get past them and just go for it.

Just as I was starting to work half-time, the bad depression came back and I felt so hopeless I wanted to die. My doc put me in the hospital and afterward kept me in the partial hospital until I fully recovered. But after going to partial all day, five days a week, it was easy to get back to half-time work at the animal shelter, and I even started taking classes again. And guess what? I'm going to get my AA degree at the end of the semester! Guess what else? I'm moving in with a friend I met at work. My mom's already planning to convert my bedroom into her "mom cave."

I hate to admit it, but you were right. When I started doing more, I found that I had more to feel happy about, and I was happier. Now I'm really excited to finally get out of this place and live like a real grownup.

Anyway, that's what made me think of writing to you, when I found your business card in my stuff while I was packing, and I just wanted to say thanks for everything.
Cheers,

Hannah 😊

Summary: Depressed Functioning
···
▶ A significant loss of function in the course of depression, or a depression that interrupts the development of normal

adult functioning—let's call it "depressed functioning"—
can lead to maladaptive habits that make it more difficult to
regain function (or for a young adult to gain it in the first
place) once the depression has ended.

▸ It may be hard in cases of depressed functioning to define
the boundaries between major depression and demoralization. There is no change in functioning to track because
the life constrictions and maladaptive habits of someone
with depressed functioning can superficially resemble the
symptoms of major depression.

▸ There is no simple way to determine whether a residual
depression is a major depressive remnant as opposed to a
lapse into depressed function. The best approach is for the
clinician to examine the patient's symptoms well beyond
the diagnostic checklist to note not only the presence or
absence of symptoms but also their quality and severity.

▸ If a clinician assumes (as I do) that the single most char-
acteristic symptom of major depressive disorder is the loss
of capacity for satisfaction, then perhaps the most telling
sign of depressed functioning is whether the person seems
to enjoy partaking in some preferred pastimes, however
limited they are in scope or ambition. Comparing two
"depressed" individuals who watch television all day long,
the person who follows a series with interest is probably
less likely to be in a major depressive episode than one who
aimlessly flips channels as a source of stimulation.

▸ Depressed functioning as a behavioral accommodation
to past major depression requires a behavioral approach
to treatment. The aims are twofold: first, to rekindle the
expectation of satisfaction in someone who, as a result of

depression, has had that expectation extinguished. Second, to extinguish the expectation that activity will be painful, by coaching the person through a gradual increase in activity.

▶ Because the boundaries between major depression and depressed functioning are indistinct, the clinician must not ignore the possibility that a change in pharmaco-therapy might also help. While engaging the patient in behavioral rehabilitation and psychotherapy, the physician can always continue to look for opportunities to improve the antidepressant response, but with the caveat that the patient is starting from a point where the antidepressants are working at least to some degree.

Case Notes

(1) The "baby blues," or postpartum sadness, is not uncom-mon and generally fades on its own. Postpartum depression is a far more serious matter. The significance of postpartum depression here may be not only the possible sign of a genetic vulnerability but also the developmental impact on Hannah of her mother's absence (and, when depressed, her mother's emotional distance) from early in Hannah's infancy.

(2) Separation and other childhood anxiety problems can be precursors of mood disorder. In Hannah's case the anxiety started so early and so consistently affected her behavior that it seems she tends toward emotional instability as a constitutional feature of her temperament rather than as an illness that changes how she reacts to stress.

(3) Habits like bulimia and self-cutting—along with kleptomania, sexual promiscuity, gambling, and other forms of reckless thrill seeking—seem to do in the depressed brain what alcohol and other substances of abuse do: they bypass the

deficit in the capacity for pleasure or satisfaction from normal activities, and thus force the reward system of the brain into action. These self-destructive behaviors may quickly become the only means a person with major depression can find to feel any relief, however transient, from the suffering of depression.

(4) Checklists should be considered only a starting point for diagnosis. Dr. Hernandez probes for more information about the symptoms than whether or not they were present. Symptom checklists without a careful follow-up interview can easily misidentify, overlook, or exaggerate symptoms. The terminology used to describe the symptoms can have different meanings to doctor and patient. Overemphasis on symptoms can occur easily, because the patient is not discouraged from rating a symptom as present even if it is explained by some other problem or is of marginal significance.

(5) Hannah's general functional inertia fuzzes the boundaries between the chronic and acute episodes of depression. Starting with a depressed level of functioning as a baseline, the deeper or darker major depressive periods can be discerned by their impact on basic activities of daily living, and on the lack of motivation to exert effort in any entertaining pastime.

(6) A psychiatrist thinking about bipolar disorder would ask whether Hannah was in fact hypomanic during the brief period after starting the antidepressant. One might guess this is not likely to be the case, however, because she had at that point already been on antidepressants for years without having any manic symptoms, and the episode resolved without further eruptions of hypomania or mood cycling. It is more likely that she was experiencing the stimulating response that sometimes occurs in the early phases of antidepressant treatment before the actual antidepressant effects start to kick in.

(7) Hannah's breakthrough depressions place her among the many individuals whose outpatient course defines their depression as treatable but high maintenance: her care will require regular visits and medication adjustments to keep her stable.

(8) Hannah's prior experiences with major depression may have left her with some residual conditioning—learned helplessness—that has impeded her adult development. Whenever she passed through a period of depression, she was conditioned during that period to expect no rewards and only negative consequences from any action on her part that required effort or risk taking. However self-defeating it is for her to go through life avoiding adult roles, it is understandable after several bouts of depression why she might feel it is not worth the effort. But the hopeful aspect of this dynamic is that it allows the possibility of reconditioning back to normal functioning once the depression is under better control.

(9) Another fairly nonstigmatizing model to explain the path from psychological invalidism back to functioning is to compare the recovery from depression to the recovery from any other major illness, or even a broken leg. After being immobilized in a cast for six weeks, a person might not expect to be at full strength immediately after the cast is removed, but rather to go through physical therapy to regain strength. After a heart attack, cardiac rehab helps restore strength and stamina to allow normal activity. Someone recovering from long or severe bouts of depression might need a similar form of rehabilitative therapy to regain the emotional stamina to withstand the normal stresses of life.

IRMA

Treatment-Refractory Depression

OVERVIEW: Irma suffers from prolonged episodes of severe, sometimes psychotic, sometimes suicidal, depression that have never entirely responded to treatment. As another episode begins, she is feeling more hopeless than ever and checks herself into the hospital. An assessment of her clinical history reveals a few treatments that have helped somewhat; electro-convulsive therapy (ECT) in particular has brought her out of the deepest depressions, but only temporarily. Although there are no "magic bullets," there are good options to consider, and a general approach to living with depression that may help keep her going until the right treatment is found or the oncoming episode resolves on its own.

"I'm here because I'm afraid I might actually do it this time. Commit suicide."

Irma is a woman in her early sixties. She was admitted Friday overnight to the psychiatric unit. Entering Irma's room is like descending into a catacomb: she has the lights off, the drapes pulled closed, the thermostat cranked low, and she's lying flat on top of the bed. Her hair is pulled back severely, and her clothing is covered by a hospital-issue bathrobe. She's fully alert, but her face betrays no hint of a social smile or pleasure to see another human being.

Dr. Imhoff is the hospital psychiatrist picking up her case Saturday morning and is meeting Irma for the first time. Irma's records are hard to find; she was previously treated on the psychiatric unit, but it was before the electronic medical record was implemented, and her paper chart is somewhere in deep storage. There's no chance the old chart will turn up before Monday. The emergency department note reveals little more than her demographics and that she has been treated for depression before, that she is suicidal, and that she cannot "contract for safety." (1)

After offering a proper introduction, Dr. Imhoff asks, "You said you were afraid you'd kill yourself 'this time'... so you have felt like killing yourself before?"

"Felt like. Tried. Repeatedly. But I always botch the job."

"And when you say you 'might actually do it,' do you mean today? Next week?"

"Not today. It's not that bad yet. But it will get worse. Then you better get out the straitjacket and throw me in the rubber room."

"Ha. We don't use those anymore, of course... but do you feel now that you need to have a nurse or an aide nearby at all times, to keep you from acting on a suicidal impulse?" Irma shakes her head no.

"Would you tell someone if you do feel that way?" Irma is quiet. Dr. Imhoff begins to wonder if she heard the question or has already forgotten it. Then Irma incants mechanically, but with reassuring eye contact: "I feel safer in the hospital, for now. I promise I will let the staff know if the urges get stronger." Encouraged by this sign of a budding therapeutic alliance, Dr. Imhoff coaxes Irma out of bed and to the office, where they sit down to do an intake interview. Given the complexity of the story and Irma's psychomotor slowing and slow speech, it could be a long interview. It is not clear that Irma is up for a long talk, so Dr. Imhoff decides to focus on gathering just the psychiatric history, for now.

Irma explains that she had been reluctant to come to the hospital, but her husband and her psychiatrist "dragged me here." Depression started to creep back into her life over the past month, after a respite of five years since her last episode. Typical of her other episodes, this one includes melancholic symptoms: despondent mood, total incapacity for desire or satisfaction, loss of interest in food, early morning awakening ("I've been awake since three a.m."), flat energy, "mental molasses," psychomotor slowing, worthlessness, suicidal urges. It was probably brought on by a change in antidepressant medications initiated a few months ago, after she complained to her outpatient psychiatrist about a low libido.

"How do you usually come out of these?" asks Dr. Imhoff.

"I don't. Nothing ever works. Just time. Lots of time."

"No treatment helps at all? But you thought the change in antidepressants caused this depression. The old one must have been doing something."

Irma looks up and sighs. "I should have said nothing works very well, or for long." She goes on, urged by steady probing questions, to describe her history with depression. She had her first serious depression after a miscarriage, when she was 21 years old. She wasn't married to the father, who was long gone by then anyway, and she wasn't getting along with her family, so she went through it alone. She had been ambivalent about having a baby at first, but she was growing to like the idea by the time of the miscarriage. After the miscarriage she felt "lower than low" and stopped showing up at work, stopped eating, stopped contacting family and friends. The idea began to take shape in her mind that she had caused the miscarriage (though her obstetrician told her otherwise), and that her miserable mood was punishment for that sin. Eventually her death, by suicide if necessary, seemed like the only way to atone. (2) Soon thereafter, a parking garage attendant found her on the top level, apparently contemplating a jump, and was able to talk her into going to the emergency department of a nearby hospital.

She was in the hospital for eight weeks that time. They first tried a tricyclic antidepressant. No help at all. Meanwhile, they had put her on an antipsychotic. "I didn't feel guilty anymore, but it made me a zombie. I could barely move." They added an anticholinergic that made her less of a "zombie," but her mood was no better. After two weeks they switched to another antidepressant. (3) "Same story. No effect at all." Four weeks into the hospital stay, looking more depressed than when she came in and still having suicidal thoughts, doctors told Irma that ECT was an option. (4) "Shock treatments. That totally freaked me out. But I didn't have a choice, really. Anyway, I was secretly hoping the shocks would kill me. I had maybe eight or nine treatments...they told me later that they thought the treatments worked, but I frankly don't remember much about it. I was still in a daze when I went home. I suppose I was better—I wasn't feeling guilty and I didn't want to kill myself and I was able to go back to work, sort of—but I wasn't back to normal, not for a long time. Maybe two years."

"And then you were back to normal?"

"Yeah, for a good six or seven years. Got married. Didn't get pregnant again, though I wanted to. My husband was infertile. Maybe that triggered the next depression, finding out we couldn't have a baby together." The second depression was remarkably like the first, but instead of feeling guilty, Irma could not shake the idea that her husband's infertility proved he had a deadly sexually transmitted disease and that she was infected, too. She thought it might be better to end her life quickly, by her own hand, than to go through the horror. "This time the shrinks didn't mess around; they went straight for the ECT. It worked—for about a month—then splat. Just as bad as before...well, not quite." Again she left the hospital, no longer delusional and not actively suicidal. She was able to work but barely, with no energy left over for any kind of social life. Her psychiatrist wanted to readmit her and resume ECT. She was determined not to go back to ECT, so instead they tried a series of outpatient medication trials.

"We tried everything—lithium, thyroid, nutritional supplements, sleep deprivation, light therapy, you name it. My psychiatrist did a fellowship at the National Institute of Mental Health and had all sorts of ideas. Even got me to do a mood chart, you know, where you rate your mood every day. That actually helped. Before that, it seemed like we made med changes based more on how I felt that day rather than how I was trending overall. But once I started doing a mood chart and bringing it to appointments, we could see whether this month was better than last month, even just a little. So if things were even a little better, we would maybe just tweak the medication, but if things were flat or declining, we knew we should make a bigger change." (5) After eighteen months, Irma was trending back toward normal on a combination of two antidepressants, lithium, and an antipsychotic medication.

"I don't know if that last combination helped or if the depression just ran its course. Either way, I felt better. Then my mother died. But actually that didn't spoil my mood at all. It probably helped, because she was a horrible narcissist."

Irma continued along a similar path up to the present. Some years would pass, and she'd feel another depression coming on despite remaining in psychiatric treatment and on meds. She would decline ECT when it was offered, and her psychiatrist would "fiddle around" with the medications until something clicked, even if it took a year or two of "fiddling." During the course of a few of these periods, she lost patience and made a suicide attempt, "but my heart was never in it. I don't know if I really wanted to die, but I didn't know what else to do. Anyway, once the suicide threat passed, I didn't feel as strong a pull to try it again." (6)

"So what's different this time?"

Irma pauses for a long time, again prompting Dr. Imhoff to wonder if she may have forgotten the question. She then says, "What's different is that my parents are both gone—my dad died last year. I was closer to him than to my mother. The thought of him finding out I'd killed myself probably kept me from doing it. My husband can take care of himself. Hell, he'd probably be relieved; I can't be very pleasant to live with. My boss and probably my shrink will feel bad if I do myself in, but they'll get over it. I can't put up with all this pain just for their sake."

"So what do you think we should do next?"

Irma looks surprised—it is the most animated facial expression she has had the whole time. "What do *I* think? You're asking me? You're the shrink—you come up with a plan, right? Nobody ever asked me what I thought before."

"I'll tell you why I asked. First, you're not psychotic; I mean, you're not delusional like you were before, when you thought you had caused your miscarriage or had contracted a sexually transmitted disease. You had the good judgment to tell someone that you weren't doing well and to sign yourself into the hospital, even though you had mixed feelings about it. So I think you are able to make an informed decision about your treatment. Second, you've had both good and bad experiences with a lot of different treatments. Some things have worked well—ECT worked for a short while, at least—and other things probably helped a little, because you weren't as depressed when you were on the right medications. Your opinions about new treatments you've heard about or about things you've tried before are an important source of information to guide us where to go from here, so again you should have a say in what we do next. The third reason is more strategic, frankly, as a way to try to steer you clear of suicide. I can see you've thought about suicide a lot. On one hand, you know the impulse has always passed, and whether or not you felt glad to be alive, you persevered. On the other hand, you're coming up with all kinds of reasons why suicide might be okay now that your parents are both gone.

"I could try to cajole you into a treatment plan. You might follow it and might even get better from it, for a while. But if you're doing treatment because I convinced you to, then the next time you are depressed and have the opportunity to commit suicide, you might take that opportunity because your interests were never an essential part of the treatment plan. No, I want you to work with us to choose your treatment so you'll be invested in it. Helping to choose your next treatment—and the one after that if necessary, and so on—would be a marker of your commitment to choose to live when you have the option to die."

Irma is quiet, but now Dr. Imhoff has no doubt that she has heard all, and is taking it in and thinking about it. "What are my options?" she murmurs. Dr. Imhoff lays out some options. "It is possible that the current medication could work or be made to work better with some dosage adjustment or augmentation. Maybe the new medication you started recently hasn't yet been brought up to a therapeutic level or had a chance to work. But that seems less likely, since you became depressed weeks after you started it, when the new medication should have already started to kick in.

"Another option would be to review the treatment history in detail, once we have all your records. We might learn there are medications and other treatment modalities you haven't tried, or tried for long enough or at high enough doses, or not tried along with augmentation strategies. Whether or not there are any obvious gaps, it is still entirely possible that a treatment that didn't work in the past might work if tried again now. You don't have the same brain you did then: it evolves.

"You've had some mixed experience with ECT, but you may

not be aware of new developments in the application of ECT that probably were not offered when you had it before. There has been a lot of new research about ways to adjust the ECT dosage—the settings—to improve the seizure quality, which can be measured routinely using brain-wave tracings, or EEG. Many people stop ECT too soon, which could explain your rapid relapses in the past. We would need to check whether your previous treatments were stopped before you were fully well, because you were a little better, or because of side effects like memory loss and confusion. If you had unilateral and never bilateral ECT, doing bilateral might be another potential to make ECT work better." (7)

"I think I did respond to ECT, but it didn't last."

"Good point. Nowadays we're doing more with mainte-nance ECT. So if you have a good response to ECT at first, then you would come back for a treatment once a week or every two weeks or every month. I've known people who stayed depression-free for years that way. With ECT spread out that much, there's little impact on memory.

"Finally, there are new things to try. Some are experimental, and some are already available but haven't yet come into general use. Transcranial magnetic stimulation, or TMS, could possibly help. It works about 50 percent of the time in some people who have treatment-resistant depression, like you, and who therefore have a low potential placebo response. Among the great advantages are that you can do it while you're doing other treatments, and it causes no cognitive side effects, so you can come in, get the treatment, and drive home. The downside is that you have to come in every day for six to eight weeks, and many insurance policies don't yet cover it. (8)

"Ketamine is still in the early phases of research, but it's out there. It's an anesthetic agent mainly, but it could give you at least a brief respite from the pain while waiting for other treatments to work. (9) There's also vagal nerve stimulation, in which you get a pacemaker put in your neck that stimulates a nerve going to your brain, but that's pretty invasive, and, like TMS, it's hit or miss in how likely it is to work. Unlike TMS, if it doesn't work, you're stuck with the apparatus in your neck. Some investigators are doing deep brain stimulation for depression—again, an electrode, this time threaded deep into your brain, and if they hit the right spot, bingo, your depression is gone. That's *if* they hit the right spot, which is the quandary at this point. They don't know if the right spot is the same spot for everyone." (10)

Irma looks a little impressed. "Wow. A lot of options. I gotta think about them."

"That's fine. Aside from ketamine and deep brain stimulation, which we don't do here, none of these things works instantly, so as long as you can assure me that you're safe—by your words and your actions—then think it through and make a choice."

Although intended as a signal to end the interview, Irma makes no move to go. "What would you choose if I were your, um, spouse?"

"I would choose the most powerful, reliable, safe treatment. That would be ECT. Granted, it's an ordeal when you're getting it, but it really works. For the longer term, I have seen with my own eyes how well maintenance ECT works for people with problems like yours. One caveat is that, thinking ahead a bit, before committing to outpatient ECT of any sort, you need a reliable means of transportation to and from treatment. You can't drive yourself home after ECT."

"My husband has to travel a lot for work, so I can't always count on him, but I do have a neighbor who would do that if I paid her a little. She's not very busy and could use the income. But what if it doesn't work—what if none of this works? Do you ever see patients with depression who get no relief from any treatment?"

Dr. Imhoff thinks momentarily. "Let's put it this way. Like most psychiatrists, I have had patients commit suicide. Short of that, I never give up. And you know what I always think about after a patient commits suicide? I think, 'If only I had more time to work with them, I know I could have found something that works.' I have seen too many people who had every reason to feel utterly hopeless come out of depression eventually. So, no, I don't think that there are any truly hopeless cases. "That being said, fighting depression when we don't know its causes, using crude tools that don't reliably help everyone, requires sort of an existential commitment to fight the good fight no matter how many times you lose. And the existential view is that feeling good is not the purpose of existence—the fight itself is the purpose."

"That doesn't sound very reassuring."

"Try looking at this this way. Before any drug is tested to see if it works on people, it is tested to see if it works on animals. How do you know if an antidepressant works in a mouse? Obviously you can't ask a mouse about its mood. The test of whether an antidepressant is likely to work in humans is whether it causes an animal to struggle longer when it is placed in a stressful situation, like being dangled by its tail or placed in a cage with more dominant animals. In these situations, an animal will always eventually surrender at some point—dangling motionless by its tail or steering clear of the alphas—but antidepressants delay the surrender. The unfortunate rodent is still hanging by its tail or bullied by the bigger rodents, but it doesn't give up as easily. The antidepressant makes it fight. So, to answer your question, there is always something else to try, even if it takes years to find it. Well, I can see I've talked too long. You're tired, and it's too much to think about right now."

"No, no, I appreciate your ideas, really. I'm leaning toward ECT, I suppose, but I still want to think about it."

"The nurses can give you some literature about the procedure, its risks, and how effective it is. And you should talk to your husband. Maybe he can be here when I see you again tomorrow, and you both can tell me then what you are thinking about treatment."

Summary: Treatment-Refractory Depression
• •

▶ Major depressive disorder is demoralizing, as it deprives a person of hope for satisfaction or relief. Antidepressant failure is even more demoralizing because the failure of treatment reinforces the hopelessness. Psychotherapy (in the form of close emotional support, theory-driven skill building, or just basic illness education) is always indicated, no matter how biologically based the major depression is thought to be. In all but the mildest cases, however, the aims of psychotherapy should be to improve coping in the here and now, and not to delve into painful past experiences. A person with major depression is impaired in the capacity to establish healthy ways to cope with old emotional injuries because of the negative bias imposed by depression, which will wane as the depression resolves through biological treatment.

▸ There are no "magic bullets." An approach that worked for one person—or even for a large majority of people—will not work for everyone. Evidence-based approaches improve the odds of success a little. An especially experienced or creative physician might further improve the odds that the next treatment intervention will be effective, but the treatment of depression is the art of knowing when and how to apply remedies discovered and tested by science.

▸ When major depression is unresponsive to treatment, then, as with any chronic disease, part of the physician's job is to maintain the person's belief that life is meaningful even while having a disease, and that there is always hope for spontaneous remission or new therapeutic developments.

Case Notes
••

(1) The "contract for safety" is a prevalent but potentially misleading clinical indicator of a person's risk for suicide. There is no evidence that a contract for safety prevents suicide or predicts a lower suicide risk. And it rests on faulty logic. A contract is by definition a mutual agreement. If one party has agreed to sacrifice something he or she professes to want, such as suicide, but ultimately perceives there is no value offered in return (in this case medical care, which for the truly suicidal person is unwanted and therefore without value), then there is nothing to keep the person from reneging on the contract. It is essential to discuss a patient's suicidal intentions, but the promise to not act on suicidal impulses is a starting point, not the endpoint, for establishing suicide risk.

Table 3. Strategies to address antidepressant failure

Modality	When to Consider	Variations	Advantages	Disadvantages
Monitoring				
Mood charting	Chronic poor treatment response, high variability of mood	Paper and pencil, smartphone app, or Web-based methods; ratings of mood, sleep, activity, and other clinical variables	Provides rich, useful data	Inconvenient, adds a burden of effort to an ill person
Medications				
Adjunctive	Partial response, limited antidepressant options	Combination antidepressants, other psychotropics, hormones, nutritional supplements	Well established, convenient, and (in some cases) supported by evidence	Increased risk of side effects
Nonstandard dosing	Poor response to standard doses, atypical or excessive side effects	Supra- and subtherapeutic doses (relative to manufacturer recommendations)	Takes into account individual variation in metabolism, sensitivity	Low evidence, increased side effect potential (with supratherapeutic dosing)
Systematic retrials	Prior trials, failure on all other classes of antidepressants	With or without augmentation by other pharmacologic and nonpharmacologic approaches	Strategy of necessity when other options exhausted, builds on past experience	Low expectations based on prior experience

Electrotherapy

ECT	Failure to respond to or to tolerate serial antidepressant medication trials; high acuity (suicide, psychosis, catatonia)	Unilateral versus bilateral; brief pulse versus ultrabrief pulse; standard six to twelve sessions versus extended course; end with maintenance or tapering versus direct transition to medication	Higher success rate than antidepressant medications	Disabling side effects during the course, temporary treatment response
TMS	Poor response to several antidepressants	Private practice versus investigational study	Minimal side effects, can be used concurrently with other therapies	High (possibly out-of-pocket) expense, limited evidence for efficacy

Referral

Psychotherapy	Demoralization complicating the presentation of or recovery from depression	Cognitive-behavioral, interpersonal, dialectical-behavioral, psychodynamic, supportive	Low risk, best way to address individual aspects of a patient's problem	Ineffective when cognitive impairment present, as in severe depression or ECT; requires large time investment by patient
Expert opinion	Complicated or atypical clinical presentation, persistent treatment nonresponse	Transition from primary care to psychiatrist, second opinion consultation, academic center	In-depth evaluation, experience-based troubleshooting	High (possibly out-of-pocket) expense, low availability
Inpatient treatment	Acute danger (psychosis, suicidality, catatonia); severe impairment; failure to respond to outpatient treatment	Community hospital (best for crisis management), tertiary referral, academic center (best for treatment refractory cases)	Assurance of safety from acute danger, safe environment for rapid treatment change, ECT, potential for fine-grained data acquisition from nursing observation	High expense, low availability

Table 4. Supplemental antidepressant treatments

Treatment Strategy	Specific Agents
Psychotropic augmentation	
Lithium	
Antiepileptics	Carbamazepine, valproate, lamotrigine
Second-generation neuroleptics	Aripiprazole, brexpiprazole, quetiapine, risperidone, etc.
Antianxiety medications	Benzodiazepines, buspirone, gabapentin
Stimulants	Dextroamphetamine, methylphenidate
Dopamine agonists	Pramipexole
Nutritional supplements	
Essential amino acids	L-tryptophan, 5-hydroxytryptophan
Omega-3 fatty acids	Fish oil
Vitamins	Folic acid (women)
Hormonal treatments	
Thyroid	Triiodothyronine (T_3), L-thyroxine (T_4)
Sexual	Dehydroepiandrosterone (DHEA), estrogen (women)
Nonpharmacological treatments	
Psychological	Cognitive behavioral therapy (CBT), interpersonal therapy (IPT), etc.
Electromagnetic	Electroconvulsive therapy (ECT), transcranial magnetic stimulation (TMS), vagus nerve stimulation (VNS)
Chronotherapy	Phototherapy (bright light therapy), sleep deprivation/phase advance

Note: Not all of these approaches are well established by evidence to be effective in general; they are listed because they have sometimes been found in clinical experience to be effective in some people.

(2) Irrational or exaggerated feelings of guilt or poverty or illness are typical "mood-congruent" delusions in people who have severe depression. Not everyone with severe major depression has such delusions, but they are an indicator of risk

for suicide or other violent acts. The fixed, false beliefs that one has committed a sin or crime, or has lost all of one's resources, or has a painful and fatal illness, are driven by the nihilistic state of mind in severe major depression, and serve to justify self-destructive acts in a vulnerable person.

(3) The general teaching is that an antidepressant may need six to eight weeks to demonstrate its full potential to resolve an episode of major depression. But within that six to eight weeks the patient and prescriber can expect to see some signs of prog-ress if the medication is likely to work, so a failure to detect any improvement at all over two weeks is a reasonable justification for switching medications early, provided there are other ready options.

(4) People commonly think of ECT as a "last resort" treatment. While it is true that ECT is more reliable than antidepressant medications at resolving major depression, and therefore a good choice when antidepressant medications haven't worked, its reliability also makes it a good choice when there is some urgency to get someone better quickly, because of either psychosis or suicidal risk or dangerously poor self-care, as in someone with catatonia.

(5) Over the long haul, when trying to build on any marginal improvement that might occur from month to month, it is essential to have consistent, fine-grained documentation of treatment response. This may come in the form of a mood chart, which can be as simple as having a patient choose a number from 1 to 10 to indicate how good or bad the mood is that day (with 1 being the utter depths of despair; 10 being elated beyond measure; and 5 being a reasonably good, steady, work-able mood). It could also be as elaborate as charting life events, symptoms, and functional indicators like duration and quality

Daily record

Sunday	Monday	Tuesday	Wednesday	Thursday	Friday	Saturday
	1	2	3	4	5	6
	3	5	5	4	4	3
7	8	9	10 *birthday!*	11	12	13
2	4	4	6	5	5	4
14	15	16	17	18	19	20

Monthly tallies

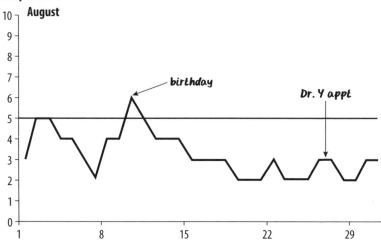

Long-term patterns

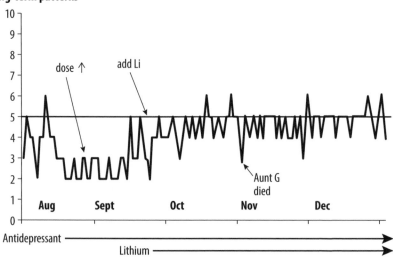

of sleep, number of work hours, social activities, panic attacks, and so on.

(6) The impermanence of suicidal intentions is another reason why a physician's job when treating depression should always be to stand in opposition to suicide. There are good data to support the assumption that someone who has attempted suicide will later be grateful that the attempt did not succeed.

(7) Specific parameters that can be measured to promote the effectiveness of ECT include the seizure quality, as measured by the postictal suppression, or the rapidity and degree of inhibition of all brainwave activity after an ECT-induced seizure. Optimizing ECT effectiveness versus its side effects involves making decisions about the use of bilateral versus unilateral treatment (bilateral being more effective, unilateral being better tolerated with regard to cognitive side effects) and

---

(*Opposite*) Daily mood recording can be as simple as jotting a number on a calendar every day. Here the scale ranges from 1 (extremely depressed) to 10 (highly manic), with 5 being a normal, everyday mood. If there is a dramatic deviation, it might help to jot down a note to explain, as this person did on the tenth of the month.

Monthly tallies use the numbers assigned to each day to give a picture of the month. It appears clear that this person's mood started to dip significantly midmonth, leading to an appointment with the psychiatrist at the end of the month. Timing matters: if the appointment with the psychiatrist had taken place around the fifteenth, fresh off the high point of the birthday and after a few days of relative stability, the low moods on the first, sixth, and seventh might have been overlooked. In context, it appears they might have been the first signs of an impending depressive phase.

Long-term patterns string together the monthly tallies to get a better gauge of treatment response. Here the dose of the antidepressant was increased in late August and seemed to have no effect until late September, when the mood started veering erratically. Lithium was added, and the average mood both rose and stabilized in the months thereafter. A blip in early November is attributable to an adverse life event.

the extension of the duration of the stimulus using ultrabrief pulses of electrical charge.

(8) TMS has been approved for use in depression. The patient, fully alert and not anaesthetized, sits up in a chair while strong magnetic pulses are administered to a carefully selected region of the left frontal lobe. The magnetic field generates an electrical current in that region of the brain. The immediate subjective effects on the patient are minimal. Over the course of weeks of regular use, some patients show persistent improvement in depressive symptoms.

(9) Ketamine is already in use as an anesthetic drug, specifically as a "dissociative" agent to induce a state of anxiety-inhibiting detachment when a patient must be kept awake for a surgical or other medical procedure. In a number of studies it has had a rapid albeit temporary antidepressant effect in a subset of people with major depression. Ketamine is also used as a recreational drug. It is a hallucinogen analogous to phencyclidine (or PCP), and it can induce a state of intoxication that might improve the mood but not permit a person to function normally while under its influence.

(10) Vagal nerve stimulation is approved as a treatment for intractable epilepsy, so it is possible to find practitioners who can legally prescribe it for depression. The most common side effect is an alteration of the voice when the device is sending an impulse. Deep brain stimulation is also being investigated for other disorders, such as Parkinson's disease, but it has proven to be effective in some people with intractable major depressive disorder. In both forms of treatment, there is a major risk: once the electrode has been placed, it can be switched off, but it is difficult if not impossible to remove it safely, regardless of whether it works.

Conclusion

To a casual observer, all nine patients in these vignettes had a sufficient number of symptoms of major depression to qualify for the diagnosis. In research protocols that rely on superficial checklist diagnostic assessments, all might have qualified for a treatment study; all but the first three cases might have qualified for a study of treatment-resistant depression. But for most of them, major depression was not the most significant active problem.

I hope stories like these demonstrate that antidepressant failure is not a simple problem like penicillin resistance, which can be addressed by merely switching to a different antibiotic. People can fail to respond, or appear to fail to respond, to antidepressants for a variety of reasons. Major depressive disorders that are, for some unknown biological reason, impervious to known or widely available biological therapies constitute a significant part of the problem, not necessarily in numbers but in the degree of suffering. A (perhaps) surprisingly large proportion of the patients I see for second or third opinions are of the sort illustrated by cases two through eight (Bob through Hannah). For these patients, biological treatments are working as well as can be expected, considering that they work poorly if at all in people who have not been taking therapeutic doses, or for whom major depressive disorder is not the only problem or who may be overmedicated.

The difficulties experienced by physicians trying to help patients like these illustrate an unfortunate reality about modern psychiatry. In every problematic case, the best treatment approach hinges on knowing detailed information about the person's life, symptoms, behavior, and constitutional vulnerabilities. This cannot be accomplished in the typical monthly fifteen- or twenty-minute "med check" visit. If you are struggling with antidepressant failure, ask your healthcare provider for more frequent or extended visits, or for a second opinion. Be sure to document and discuss the details about the quality, context, duration, course, and intensity of your symptoms, and how they specifically affect your functioning. Also, you should involve family or partners in your meetings with your care provider; people close to you can provide a richer basis for your provider to understand the differences between good and bad times. The additional information to be gained from longer and more frequent visits, from second opinions, or from additional informants, as illustrated by some of the patients portrayed in this book, can make a critical difference in developing a more effective approach to treatment.

Appendix A
Assessment of Antidepressant Failure

Success in treating the depressed patient who has not
responded to antidepressants hinges on knowing what kind of
depression the person has: major depressive disorder, demoralization, depressed functioning, a depressive personality, or
some combination of these. Thorough history taking informed
by a few key questions can help to untangle what experiences,
dispositions, and behaviors block a person's therapeutic
response to antidepressants.

Major Depressive Disorder

For a person who comes to see a physician with the problem
of antidepressant failure, prior diagnosis of major depressive
disorder is almost always a given, so the interviewer's aim is to
confirm or question it. The gold standard for diagnosis is the
description of a sufficient number of designated symptoms,
at sufficient severity for a minimum duration, and not better
explained by other clinical factors. Diagnostic certainty can be
hard to achieve even with a lucid patient using a structured
interview, however. Establishing an unequivocal diagnosis in
the absence of vivid symptom descriptions may entail some
creative reasoning.

- ▶ Did the person really have major depressive disorder in the
  past?
  - ▷ Some patients may be able to recall the specific symp-
    toms of a past episode, but many will not. A past medical

record that documents the symptoms active at the time is perhaps the best evidence. A history of gross fluctuations in functioning—leaves of absence from work or school, periods of discontinuation from social activity, suicidal crises—may support the diagnosis without fully proving it. If there is still scanty evidence that past episodes really were major depressive episodes, then the physician might ask how the diagnosis was assigned. Can the patient explain why a physician in the past thought the patient had major depression?

▶ Does the person currently have major depressive disorder?

▷ Before assuming that antidepressants have failed and that a new medication strategy is needed, ongoing symptoms of depression should satisfy the minimal criteria for severity that have been established as reliable indicators of the presence of major depressive disorder. The task is to determine the quality of a person's symptoms and tie them specifically to functional impact. ("You said you had to stop working. Was it because you had too little energy, or motivation, or inability to focus, or something else?") If the functional impact of depressive symptoms remains equivocal, it increases the likelihood that they are symptoms of something other than major depressive disorder.

▶ Are the person's symptoms of major depressive disorder better explained by some other condition, like delirium or bipolar disorder?

▷ Because the patient (and presumably the referring physician) assumes the problem to be major depressive disorder, a consultant will likely need to probe specifically to rule out alterations in consciousness on one hand, and periods of mania or hypomania on the other.

- An assessment of an overly sleepy, agitated, or fluctuating level of arousal, or a description of altered level of arousal by other informants, would support a diagnosis of delirium.

- Querying whether the person has had periods of elevated, excited, or extremely irritable mood; high or restless energy; diminished need to sleep; rapid thoughts; or inflated self-attitude would elicit a determination of bipolar disorder. Not everyone who has ever been too excited to sleep has bipolar disorder, of course, but generally only someone with bipolar disorder or on stimulating medications would be able to avoid sleep for several days running.

Assuming the diagnosis is not in question, the most crucial information needed to inform the next antidepressant trial is a thorough treatment history. A simple list of past medication trials may not be all that useful; the physician would like to be able to determine not only which drugs the patient took, but also whether the trial of each drug was adequate to determine that the drug did not work. If any trials were cut short by side effects, then find out enough about the side effects to be reasonably certain that they were caused by the antidepressant in question.

If there is sufficient time, memory, and documentation, the physician can lay out a timeline from the onset of illness to the present, year by year, plotting out when the patient had depressions, when, if ever, the patient was depression-free, and when there were major life events that may have influenced the clinical picture at the time. Adjacent to that timeline, the physician can then indicate the intervals of time during which the patient was treated with each medication in the history. If (as is often the case) there were many such medications, a detailed timeline may be the only way to observe the benefits, or lack thereof, of combination trials.

Periods of nontreatment may be as important as treatment episodes in understanding patterns of treatment response. When collapsing a life history into a brief interview, it is easy for both patient and physician to lose sight of patterns that occurred during otherwise uneventful periods. It can be just as important to know how frequently or intensely a person's depressive disorder worsened when not taking medications as it is to know whether he or she responded to a given medication. A chronically depressed person thus might not otherwise notice that there was a long period while on a given antidepressant when the mood never reverted to happy, but there were few or no severe episodes. A person with rapid mood fluctuations might not readily perceive that the period since antidepressant treatment began has actually been worse (suggestive of an underlying, subtle bipolar spectrum disorder exacerbated by antidepressant use).

Demoralization

If a person is demoralized but does not have major depressive disorder, then antidepressants are unlikely to lift the mood; if a person is demoralized on top of having major depressive disorder, the therapeutic response to antidepressants may be muted. Whichever the case, the key to alleviating demoralization is to change the patient's outlook. So the clinician begins by understanding how the patient views the situation as it stands. Because the patient's view can evolve day by day, with every new experience, the clinician's role may also require an ongoing therapeutic relationship in order to keep up.

In cases where the careful review of major depressive symptoms illustrated above leaves some room to doubt that the patient currently has a major depressive disorder, it may be fruitful to switch to some projective questioning, on the assumption that a person in the grip of a major depressive disorder will have an impaired capacity not only to experience pleasure and satisfaction but also to imagine or anticipate them. The interviewer might ask a question like this: "Suppose I had a new drug that would take away your depression by tomorrow morning. How would you spend your tomorrow? Next month? Next year?" Neither a truly depressed nor simply demoralized person will likely respond with a robust itinerary, but with some coaxing the demoralized person without major depression should be able to identify things he or she would like to do (if only the demoralizing situation could be resolved). People with major depressive disorder have a hard time with this question because they have lost the capacity to anticipate pleasure and satisfaction.

Hopelessness and helplessness are often the hallmarks of demoralization when it occurs on top of major depressive disorder. These symptoms are not essential symptoms of major depressive disorder; many individuals can have major depression without hopelessness, as they know it will eventually resolve, and also without helplessness, as they know treatment is available. Understanding a patient's hopelessness or helplessness can begin with a simple question, like "What would successful treatment for your depression look like?" Such a question induces a patient to amplify on whatever hope there is for recovery, and whatever trust there is in treatment.

Depressed Functioning

Although the differences may be subtle, a poorly functioning person with major depressive disorder can be differentiated from a poorly functioning person who never had or has recovered from major depressive disorder, on the basis of a close reading of symptoms—which in depressed functioning will be mild-moderate in severity—and day-to-day activities. Starting with when and how the patient arises from sleep, the physician should discuss the essential activities of daily living, finding out when and how (and how often) the patient is able to accomplish them. End with documenting the hours the patient goes to bed and when the patient falls asleep. Go into detail. If the patient spends much of the day in bed or on the couch, find out what he or she does while recumbent. Excessive sleeping, aimless channel flipping, staring vacantly at the ceiling all support a diagnosis of major depressive disorder. Motivated television watching, reading Russian novels, blogging throughout the day every day suggest a person who, although sedentary, has not lost interest in activities and who may not have major depressive illness.

Depressive Personality

In contrast to someone with depressed functioning, who functions at a lower level than might be predicted given the mild-moderate severity of depressive symptoms, a person with depressive personality is likely to function better than might be expected, given the persistence of mild-moderate depressive symptoms. A person with depressive symptoms might function better than expected for one of two reasons: either the person has remarkable resilience that allows the maintenance of good functioning despite having a major depressive disorder, or the major depressive disorder is not sufficiently severe to cause role dysfunction and therefore could not be formally considered a major depressive disorder that would likely respond to antidepressant therapy. The person in the latter case might have a depressive personality that affects the enjoyment of life without affecting the capacity to perform life roles. This conclusion should only be reached once the clinician is fully satisfied that major depression is not an active problem.

Perhaps the strongest positive evidence that a chronically depressed, antidepressant-insensitive person might have a depressive personality that mimics major depressive disorder can be derived from the ability or inability to identify *any* period when the person was reasonably satisfied and enjoying life. One can start by asking, "When was the last time you were feeling well?" A person with major depressive disorder might not be able to enjoy recalling past good times but should at least be able to recall that there were such times before the major depression hit. A person with a depressive predisposition, in contrast, is more likely to respond with something like "never."

Appendix B
Common Therapeutic Practices to Boost Antidepressant Response

When a person with major depressive disorder has clearly not had adequate benefit from antidepressant treatment, what can one do? The strategies available can roughly be summarized as switching and combining. Note that these approaches are largely informed by evidence but are not limited to evidence-based approaches that have been vetted by controlled clinical trials.

When to Switch Antidepressants

The standard teaching is that an antidepressant trial requires six to eight weeks at a therapeutic dose to realize its full potential to resolve a major depressive episode.

Under some circumstances, it makes sense not to wait the full six to eight weeks:

- ▶ There is no sign whatsoever of symptom improvement after two weeks of treatment.
- ▶ An intolerable or medically deleterious side effect occurs early in the course of treatment.
- ▶ The patient has a rapid worsening of illness toward psychosis, suicidality, or catatonia that warrants immediate electroconvulsive therapy (ECT).

Extending the trial beyond the six to eight weeks may be reasonable in other circumstances:

- ▶ Symptoms have continued to improve gradually throughout the six- to eight-week period.

▶ The patient can still safely tolerate an increased dosage; therefore the trial may be continued at a higher dosage.

▶ External factors that might have inhibited medication response, such as concurrent alcoholism or drug abuse, can be addressed.

▶ There are few other antidepressant options to explore or many untried augmentation or combination strategies.

How to Switch Antidepressants

Points to keep in mind when replacing an ineffective antidepressant:

▶ Consider switching antidepressant types; for example, before trying a third selective serotonin reuptake inhibitor (SSRI), consider a serotonin-norepinephrine reuptake inhibitor (SNRI).

▶ Look for potentially beneficial side effects:
  ▷ If a patient is not eating or sleeping well, try a drug with sedating and appetite-enhancing qualities, like mirtazapine.
  ▷ If a patient has problems with chronic pain, consider an SNRI or tricyclic antidepressant (TCA).
  ▷ If a patient is mostly concerned with poor concentration or lethargy, consider an activating medication, such as bupropion.
  ▷ Don't be limited by purported side effects, however. If an activating antidepressant raises anxiety in the short term but might ultimately defeat the cause of anxiety by alleviating depression, then it should be considered.

▶ Consider older antidepressants—although harder to use, they have advantages:

▷ TCA therapeutic blood levels can be measured, so dosage can be precisely titrated.

▷ Physicians often overlook monoamine oxidase inhibitors (MAOIs) because of the potential for food and drug interactions, but they are uniquely beneficial in a subset of patients.

When making the switch, consider the opportunity to conduct a trial of combination antidepressant therapy in the process.

► Combination antidepressant treatment can be tested as an option while cross tapering to an antidepressant drug in a different class.

► Cross tapering or combination treatment should be conducted at a slower pace than a direct switch, both because of the potential for deleterious drug interactions and in order to gauge the potentially synergistic effects of the combination before withdrawing the first agent.

Combinations

Antidepressant-Antidepressant Combinations

Data do not provide much support for the efficacy of combinations of two or more antidepressants, compared to using a single antidepressant. There are circumstances in which a physician might favor a two-antidepressant approach, including:

► During a crossover from one antidepressant to another, the patient has a remarkably good early result while on both agents.

► A second antidepressant adds a beneficial side effect; for example, trazodone provides nocturnal sedation to a person with depression and insomnia taking a nonsedating antidepressant.

Antidepressant–Other Drug Combinations

A wide variety of agents have been combined with antidepressants, ranging from neuroleptics and lithium to hormonal and nutritional supplementation.

▶ *Lithium* (which is an effective but seldom-used antidepressant in its own right) has consistently demonstrated strong evidence of efficacy in combination with antidepressants at augmenting an inadequate antidepressant response. There is also evidence that lithium in combination with an antidepressant can substantially improve the duration of recovery after resolution of depression using ECT. Although lithium's narrow therapeutic window makes it difficult to use—blood tests are required to ensure that the patient is on the correct dose, and to monitor for diminished thyroid and renal function—when used as a combination therapy, one can aim for the safer, low end of the therapeutic range, approximately 0.6 to 0.8 mEq/L.

▶ Some *neuroleptics*, in low doses, have activating pharmacologic effects aside from dopamine blockade; these drugs include (but are not limited to) fluphenazine, aripiprazole, brexpiprazole, and risperidone. Among these, aripiprazole and brexpiprazole have approval from the US Food and Drug Administration for use as augmentation strategies for treatment-resistant depression. Most neuroleptics, at low to moderate doses, have tranquilizing effects sufficient to improve anxiety and agitation in a person with anxious or agitated depression, and to induce sleep in a depressed person with insomnia.

- Others:
  - *Low-dose thyroid hormone* (triiodothyronine, or T3) is a fairly benign and, in the view of some, effective strategy to boost a poor antidepressant response. There is some evidence to suggest that it is most effective in people who do not have a thyroid abnormality and whose thyroid levels are in the low range of normal (i.e., high-normal thyroid-stimulating hormone, or TSH).
  - *Antiepileptics* with efficacy in bipolar disorder have also been found to be successful as add-on treatments to antidepressants; these include lamotrigine, carbamazepine, and valproic acid. Gabapentin, topiramate, and phenytoin have questionable, if any, utility in bipolar disorder and have not proven helpful in combination antidepressant therapy.
  - *Pramipexole*, a dopamine agonist, is an effective albeit higher-risk augmentation strategy for major depressive disorder.
  - *Buspirone* has been shown in at least one randomized placebo-controlled clinical trial to boost SSRI response in treatment-resistant depression.
  - Pharmacologic enhancement of *gonadal steroids* in combination with antidepressants is associated with improved outcome, but the benefit seems limited to patients who have abnormal hormonal function.
  - *Nutritional supplementation* with L-tryptophan, folic acid, S-adenosyl methionine, and omega-3 fatty acids is a low-risk strategy supported by a modicum of evidence to enhance antidepressant response.

Antidepressant-Nonpharmacologic Combinations

Psychotherapy

Treatment-resistant major depression is highly demoralizing—not only do sufferers feel the agony of the depressive illness itself, but they also must contend with the discouraging fact that asking for help and accepting treatment did not provide relief. Education and support in the form of psychotherapy enhance the response to antidepressants by alleviating the sense of helplessness.

The secondary role of psychotherapy addresses the predisposing and residual factors that contribute to or result from a major depressive episode. The mode of therapy can be matched to the patient's specific problem. Behavioral rehabilitation helps to bridge the gap from remission to functional recovery. Cognitive behavioral therapy (CBT) for a person who has recovered from depression extinguishes maladaptive attitudes learned in the course of depression. Interpersonal therapy on maintenance antidepressant treatment may help prevent recurrence by improving a person's relationships with supportive others.

Electrotherapy

Pharmacotherapy at the same time as *electroconvulsive therapy* warrants caution, as almost any psychoactive substance can potentiate the cognitive side effects from ECT. Bupropion, in particular, must be avoided concurrently with ECT, as it may increase the risk of an uncontrolled seizure. Antidepressants might be used concurrently with a tapering or maintenance course of ECT, however, where the risk of cognitive side effects is lower. In contrast, there are no contraindications to using antidepressant medications in combination with *transcranial magnetic stimulation* (TMS), so for a person with treatment-resistant depression, a trial of TMS need not interfere with ongoing pharmacotherapeutic trials.

Index

Page numbers in italics refer to figures and tables.